Published by Word Therapy Publishing
November 15, 2016

ISBN-13: 978-0975516324

ISBN-10: 0975516329

Cover Design by: Cordelia Gaffar

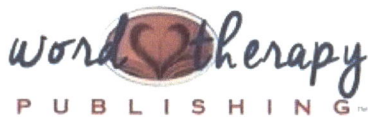

word therapy
P U B L I S H I N G™

Word Therapy Publishing
P.O. Box 939
Hope Mills, NC 28348
www.wordtherapypublishing.com
888-494-8880

Dedication

With immense gratitude and appreciation, I am humbled by the patience and love
husband Riad and the cooking assistance and artistic expertise of my three older children
Ameenah, Muhibbah and Humdan.

This book serves as the second edition of my first book, **The Guide: How to Get Started with Workout Around My Day**. Much of the beginning chapters are the same, however, many chapters have been added. There is now a whole section dedicated for self-nurturing and a recipe book.

DISCLAIMER AND TERMS OF USE AGREEMENT

The author and publisher have used their best efforts in preparing this guide. The author and publisher make no representation or warranties with respect to the accuracy, applicability, fitness, or completeness of the contents of this report. The information contained in this guide is strictly for educational purposes. Therefore, if you wish to apply ideas contained in this report, you are taking full responsibility for your actions.

Every effort has been made to accurately represent this product and its potential. However, there is no guarantee that you will improve in any way using the techniques and ideas in this guide, with the audio workouts or any other accompanying products. Examples of success with this product should not be interpreted as a guarantee.

Your level of improvement in attaining the results claimed in the materials depends on the time and effort you devote to the program, ideas and techniques mentioned, knowledge and various skills. Since these factors differ per individuals, we cannot guarantee your success or improvement level. Nor are we responsible for any of your actions.

Many factors will be important in determining your actual results and no guaranteed are made that you will achieve results like ours or anybody else's, in fact no guarantees are made that will achieve any results from our ideas and techniques.

The author and publisher disclaim any warranties (express or implied), merchantability, or fitness for any purpose. The author and publisher shall in no event be held liable to any party for any direct, indirect, punitive, special, incidental or other consequential damages arising directly or indirectly from any use of this material, which is provided "as is", and without warranties.

As always, the advice of a competent professional should be sought.

The author and publisher do not warrant the performance, effectiveness or applicability of any sites listed or linked to in this report. All links are for information purposes only and are not warranted for content, accuracy or any other implied or explicit purpose.

as brief quotations or as prescribed by the program instructions without the written permission of the publisher.

Workout Around My Day Inc., P.O. Box 1396, Charles Town, WV 25414

cordelia@workoutaroundmyday.com

Contents

My Story: A Journey Towards Health and Fitness

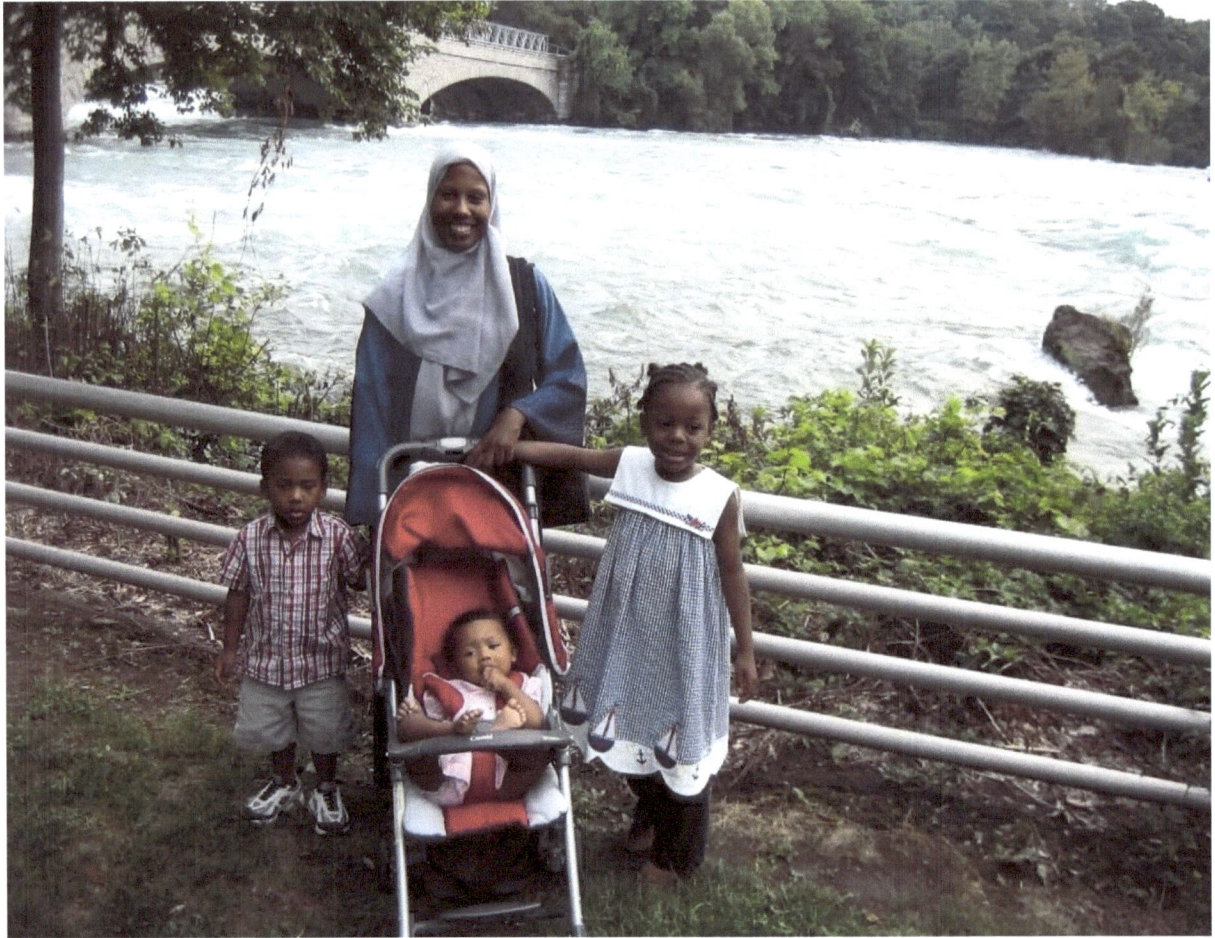

Niagara Falls 2005

About 15 years ago, after my oldest was born, I worked full-time. Whoa, life changed. Juggling husband, home, hearth, new baby and working outside the home, I lost myself to a new rhythm sung off-key. Determined not to become an overwhelmed new mommy, I made me-time early in the morning before the rest of the house stirred. Each day I would exercise before breakfast, before work, before drop off to daycare, often for a good 25 minutes watching a full workout video. Staying in shape pushed me to use the stairs at work (up and down nine floors at least three times a day, I might add). At lunchtime, I hit the stairs both ways before and after a yummy meal I either brought from home, or picked up from a trusted vendor. On good days, I would do a few laps around the track during and after lunch. Most evenings, if my energy kicked in, I would do jumping jacks and push-ups or something callisthenic just to recharge and have enough energy for dinner, my child's bedtime routine, etc. By the end of the day, after having worked out so much, I needed to stretch.

What was so remarkable is this all happened very naturally. I needed Me-time to recharge and release the stress of the day. I wasn't anxious to lose excess baby weight. In fact, I had returned to my pre-pregnancy size in the immediate six weeks following delivery by simply nursing. The need to nourish and replenish myself to care for my family helped me establish early fitness habits that organically grew into greater knowledge about fitness and nutrition.

With my second child, though, it was a completely different story. After I had my son, for the first time in my life, I was weak, tired and fat. Walking hurt and my "baby belly" did not melt away with nursing. I was panicked! OMG, will I look like this forever? Is this what they mean when they said that you lose your shape and beauty after pregnancy? The mental negative talk started.

My downward spiral stopped by me realizing that my grandmother had five children and remained petite. My mother also had four children and stayed petite. So genetically, I was not doomed. Just a side bar about genetics, there is no such thing as being 'genetically doomed'. Research shows that all things can be overcome nutritionally and by changing your habits. Per an article on Psychologytoday.com, "A recently reported analysis of studies on an obesity gene, FTO, has concluded that if obesity "runs in the family" then running will prevent the family from becoming obese. The study suggests if all your relatives on both sides of your family can't see their laps when they sit down, if you run or otherwise engage in physical activity, it is doubtful that you will be fat."[1] Moreover, in more recent studies on the FTO gene in Sweden and London, the conclusion reached stated, "genetic factors are to blame only for about five percent of all cases."[2] **Back to my story**. After my first pregnancy, I made a schedule to fit in workouts throughout my day. However, this was far more challenging the second time around because there never seemed to be the "right" time to do it. I no longer had time to watch a full video, and baby boy awoke almost as soon as I would get into my morning workout. The most I could get in were 5 to 10 minutes at a time.

, [1] "Can Your Genes Really Make You Fat?", November 7, 2011, www.psychologytoday.com
[2] "Do Your Genes Make You Fat?" Q&A on www.drweil.com, November 8, 2013

Researching the most time compounding exercises with the best results led me to Pilates. It promised a feminine physique and the benefits of weight lifting without the bulk. The shortest beginner's video I found was 25 minutes. I did what I could in my 5 to 10- minute window. Three weeks into my new exercise routine, the results shocked me. I had lost my belly even though most days I had only done the 25-minute video in sections of 5 or 10 minutes during my day. At that point, I decided to try to memorize the routine and continue using it in sections whenever I could fit it in. On weekend mornings, I was able do the entire video.

Eventually I chose staying home (part-time working from home) with my children over going into an office each day, so my midday workouts became running up and down the stairs as I did my housework. Working from my home-office meant mommy-duty, too. Caring for children is a workout itself; but the video routines worked wonders. I maximized my results for effort and time I put in with Pilates. Stretching, body resistance, and strengthening exercises left me with sleek and toned results. At the end of six months, I found that I was back to my pre-pregnancy physique. I made up my own routine before dinner for an evening recharge and then again before sleep.

After the third baby, I jumped right back to square one. The clock was ticking and my body was losing its battle with blubber. Aside from chasing my kids at the playground, or on their bikes/ trikes, I did not exercise during this pregnancy. Although Pilates offers strengthening and body resistance, I found I needed an actual weight-bearing workout. I lost the weight but had some sag and needed to preserve muscle tone. And then there was the fact that things did not stay in place for long. If I missed a day of exercise, I jiggled in all the wrong places, if you know what I mean. I began researching what to do to keep away the sag. Who wants to *NEED* to wear Spanx?

I was back to a morning 20- to 25-minute workout with weights and then several 5 to 10-minute sessions throughout the day. The weights routine in the morning had another awesome effect…it made me super energetic even without a cup of coffee! A bonus…experts recommended heavy protein meals to rebuild and feed those ripping muscles. Yum!

When I think back on my journey, I notice a specific set of habits that now form the basis of my wellness program. These experiences helped me establish a method to work out around my day. After my fourth, fifth, and now sixth child, I have been further able to develop my program and enhance it with continued research.

Today, I don't struggle to return to my former weight and body. I can consistently achieve and maintain incredible results because of the simple habits I learned to establish and practice every day. Little shifts in my food choices, short workouts throughout the day, and targeted exercise did the trick. That is my story, and in the next pages, I will share the secrets of how you too can accomplish healthy weight and nutrition goals that fit around your day.

The Workout Around My Day method has taken me years to perfect. I have written this book to give you its benefits in just a few pages. I begin by giving you some background on food choices and tips on how new ones can easily be integrated into your routine. Next, I will show you how your movements can be modified to strengthen your body. Finally, we will get to the details of scheduling workouts into your day. At this point, it will be your turn to reflect on your eating, movements and scheduling and modify each gradually over the period of 5 days for each new system. Congratulations on starting on your path to self-nurturing!

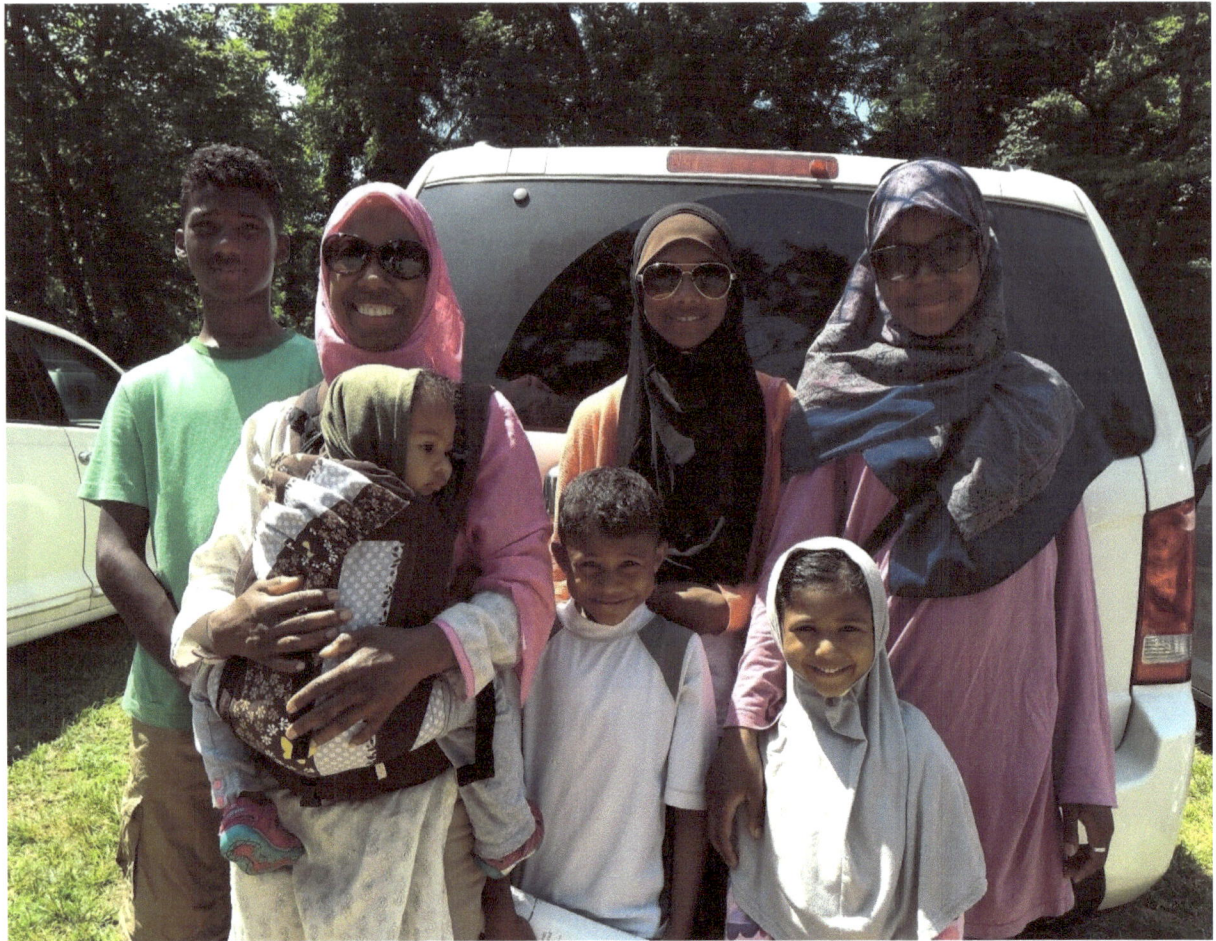

Field Trip June 2016 (left to right Humdan, me and Arlene, back row Muhibbah (baby in the stroller in previous picture), Ameenah, Imran and Muniba)

The Power of Food Choices

I know many of us struggle to eat healthy. My parents, though, were powerful influences in how I learned to make the right food choices, and I credit them for providing me with a foundation that has lasted into my adulthood. I remember eating the harvest of my mother's kitchen garden and having our largest meal early in the day. As a teen, I traveled to France and adopted the French practice of eating smaller meals as the day progressed, which was new to me.

Here I will show you how to make powerful food choices, adjust meal portions, and time your meals just right.

First, though, I want you to consider the challenges we face in achieving an ideal diet:

- Maintaining optimal hydration
- Managing energy level and food cravings
- Finding the best time for meals

To address these challenges, I have discovered a few simple fixes:

1. Start adding hydrating fruits and vegetables to your diet.
2. Choose slow energy-releasing foods and limit sugary snacks.
3. Do not eat once the sun goes down.

First, let's address hydration. The reality is some of our preferred beverages will just bring us down. You know the ones: carbonated thirst-quenchers, juices, alcohol and sweet drinks. I would replace them with coconut water and coconut water homemade mixes. Juicing is always an option too. While these are great alternatives, water is always the best beverage, but not everyone can drink the appropriate quantity. I've found a great way to boost your daily water intake. Make popsicles by adding berries or other favorite fruit to your water and freeze them. You can also have a cup of water before each meal and immediately following. If you eat at least three times a day that is six glasses already. Add a glass of water before any snacks or instead of a morning and afternoon snack and you are up to 8 cups. The body needs about ½ an ounce of water for every pound you weigh or 1 ounce per kg.

Before I discuss hydrating fruits and vegetables, you need to understand that not all produce is created equal. This list is compiled and released each spring around April or May on ewg.org. The website is a very useful resource for skin care, hair care and household products as well. The Dirty Dozen and Clean 15, lists compiled by the Environmental Working Group (EWG), help explain this issue:

> [T]he Dirty Dozen is an invaluable aid to helping decide which of the fruits and vegetables we purchase should be organic. The Clean list 15 provides us with information about what produce contains the least amount of pesticide residues. This year the "Dirty Dozen Plus" category highlights hot peppers, kale, and collard greens. Per the EWG, these vegetables "did not meet traditional Dirty Dozen criteria but were commonly contaminated with highly toxic organophosphate insecticides. These insecticides are toxic to the nervous system and have been largely removed from agriculture over the past decade. But they are not banned and still show up on some food crops."

Slow energy-releasing food examples include: whole grains, fruits, vegetables and legumes. This is where it is important to understand portion size. On the web site heart.org[3], there is a quiz where you can test your knowledge on a proper serving size. See below:

Which food on the left matches the portion size on the right?

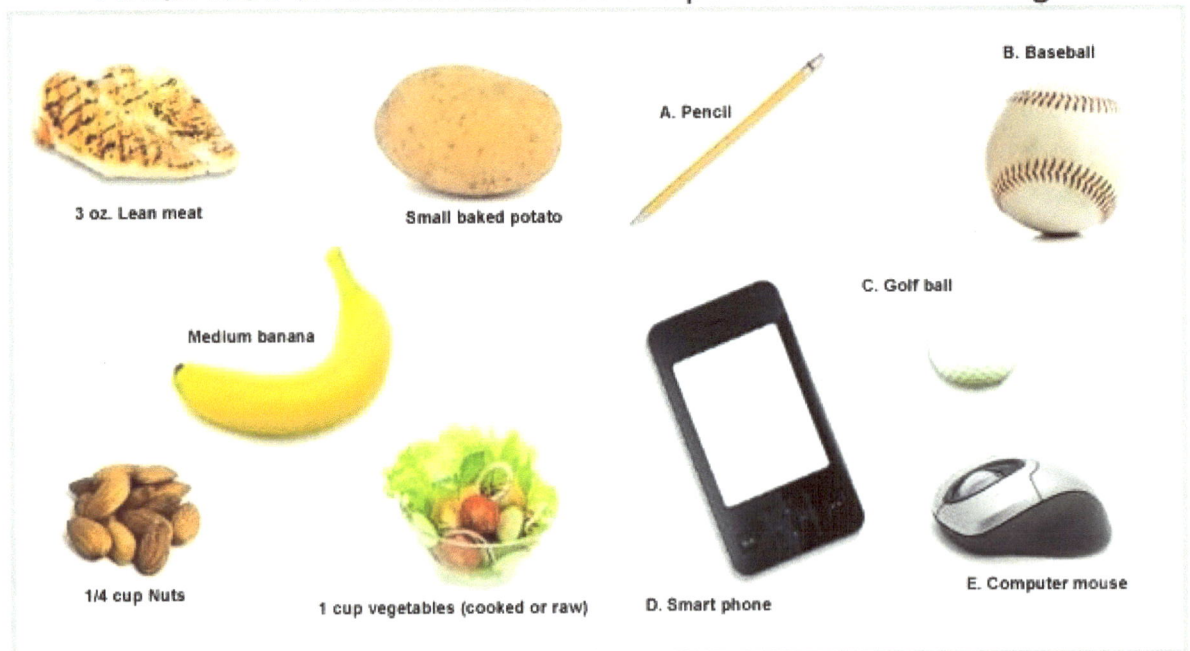

3 oz. Lean meat

Small baked potato

A. Pencil

B. Baseball

Medium banana

C. Golf ball

D. Smart phone

E. Computer mouse

1/4 cup Nuts

1 cup vegetables (cooked or raw)

[3] Heart.org http://www.heart.org/ from article called "Portion Size versus Serving Size" and "Don't Fall Prey to Portion Distortion"

You may be surprised to learn these are serving sizes:

- 1 slice of bread
- ½ cup rice or pasta (cooked)
- 1 small piece of fruit (super-large apples are 2+ servings)
- 1 wedge of melon
- ¾ cup fruit juice
- =1 cup milk or yogurt
- 2 oz. cheese (about the size of a domino)
- 2-3 oz. meat, poultry or fish (this is about the size of a deck of cards)

In general, "think small fist, baseball, hockey puck and a computer mouse. These are all things that describe a "serving size." The comparisons will help you eat more of the things you need and less of the things you don't.

- One serving of raw leafy vegetables or a baked potato **should be about the size of a small fist**. A serving is a lot smaller than most people think.
- A cup of fat-free or low-fat milk or yogurt, or a medium fruit should **equal about the size of a baseball**.
- A half a bagel is about the **size of a hockey puck** and represents a serving from the grains group.
- Three ounces of cooked lean meat or poultry is about the **size of a computer mouse**. Three ounces of grilled fish is about the **size of a checkbook**.
- A teaspoon of soft margarine is about the **size of one die**.
- An ounce of fat-free or low-fat cheese is about the **size of six stacked dice**.

Whole Grains: Red, brown or parboiled rice, rolled oats, bulgur

Fruits: In season choices are always best. Winter (December – February): grapefruit, oranges, tangerines, dates, red bananas, kiwi; Spring (March – May): apricots, jackfruit; Summer (June – August): most berries, melons, peaches, nectarines; Fall (September – November): pomegranate, grapefruit, grapes, guava. For full list see http://www.nourishinteractive.com/.

Dried fruits and berries are also an option: goji, golden, dates, and figs.

Vegetables: In season choices are always best. See http://www.nourishinteractive.com/ for a complete list.

Legumes: A legume is a fruit or vegetable from the pea family. Some common examples are alfalfa, beans, lentils, peanuts and tamarind.

Some nuts and seeds that are also slow releasing sugar balancing plant proteins are: hemp, sunflower, chia, flax, pumpkin, pistachios, almonds, walnut.

Low IG _glycemic level also needs to be considered:

Fruits: Apple, Pear, Peach, dates, grapefruit, prunes (also see Dirty dozen for organic recommendations) Vegetables: yam, beans, parsnips, sweet potatoes (also see Dirty dozen for organic recommendations)

Try this Seven Day Portion Control Challenge

Here are the terms of the seven- day challenge:

- **Use a smaller plate, 8 in diameter or a salad size plate**
- **Fill it with fresh in season fruits and/ or vegetables, a protein, a small piece or bread or ½ cup of rice or pasta**
- **Sit up straight and chew your food at least 15 times before swallowing**
- **Drink a full glass of water upon completion**
- **Journal your results: feeling full or feeling empty**

Below is a picture of what your plate should look like.

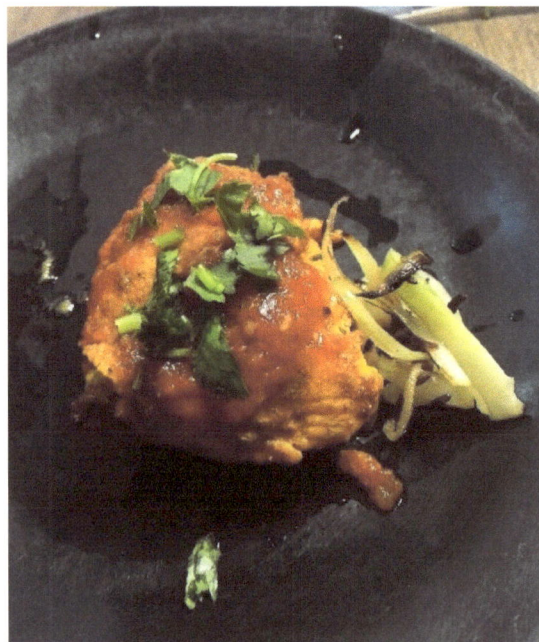

Adult size portion of salmon over sweet potato

Implementation Log:

Today:

_____
_____
_____
_____

Morning ___ Satisfied___ Hungry___ No Change

_____
_____
_____
_____

Afternoon ___ Satisfied___ Hungry___ No Change

_____
_____
_____
_____

Evening ___ Satisfied___ Hungry___ No Change

Day 2:

_____
_____
_____
_____

Morning ___ Satisfied___ Hungry___ No Change

_____
_____
_____
_____

Afternoon ___ Satisfied___ Hungry___ No Change

_____
_____
_____
_____

Evening ___ Satisfied___ Hungry___ No Change

Day 3:

_____

Morning ___ Satisfied___ Hungry___ No Change

_____

Afternoon ___ Satisfied___ Hungry___ No Change

_____

Evening ___ Satisfied___ Hungry___ No Change

Day 4:

Morning ___ Satisfied___ Hungry___ No Change

Afternoon ___ Satisfied___ Hungry___ No Change

Evening ___ Satisfied___ Hungry___ No Change

Day 5:

_____
_____
_____
_____

Morning ___ Satisfied___ Hungry___ No Change

_____
_____
_____
_____

Afternoon ___ Satisfied___ Hungry___ No Change

_____
_____
_____
_____

Evening ___ Satisfied___ Hungry___ No Change

Day 6:

_____
_____
_____
_____

Morning ___ Satisfied___ Hungry___ No Change

_____
_____
_____
_____

Afternoon ___ Satisfied___ Hungry___ No Change

_____
_____
_____
_____

Evening ___ Satisfied___ Hungry___ No Change

Day 7:

_____
_____
_____
_____

Morning ___ Satisfied___ Hungry___ No Change

_____
_____
_____
_____

Afternoon ___ Satisfied___ Hungry___ No Change

_____
_____
_____
_____

Evening ___ Satisfied___ Hungry___ No Change

Making Better Selections

I believe that we should weigh our purchasing options and in turn our purchasing power. There is so much information today about what is 'good' for us. However, to better understand what our bodies need we must start from our humble beginnings. Humans made choices based on in-season availability. Seeds, berries and leaves were available most of the year. Then we learned how to hunt for meat. Again, only certain animals were available at certain times. Even when we learned to domesticate fowl and other animals, we used their milk or eggs and could not always eat them. Today, any type of meat, seeds, fruits and leaves are available year-round. But take time to tune into what produce or meat is cheaper and when. This is the key to in-season foods. Better yet, shop at the farmer's market, specialty health food store, or join a CSA (community support agriculture). In the previous section, we also touched on resources for in-season produce.

Next, adjust your food selection, eating and cooking practices accordingly. You will notice that using simple whole food selections will bring you more energy, better health and mental clarity. Notice the recommended state of food. You should be inclined to go against genetically modified foods and against poisoning our children with deadly toxins. The ancient art of eating foods in season and eating for health has been gradually stolen from humanity with the dawn of industrialization, which spawned greed. If we grow what we need and eat what is in season instead of growing more than we need, we could solve 60% of common health issues. For example, dandelion leaves are a great source of calcium, iron, and vitamins A – K.

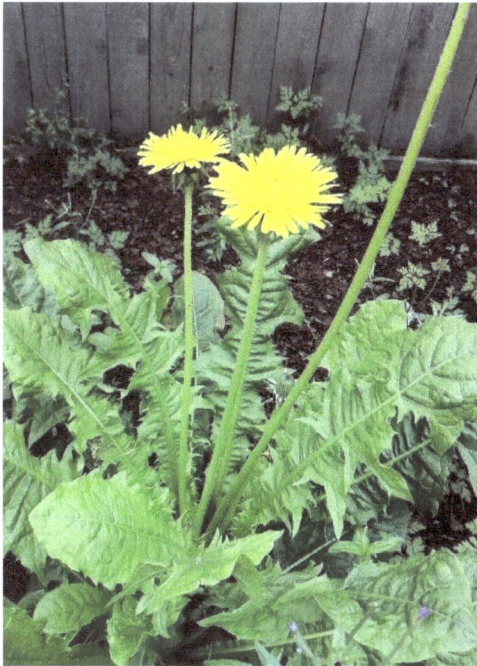
Dandelion

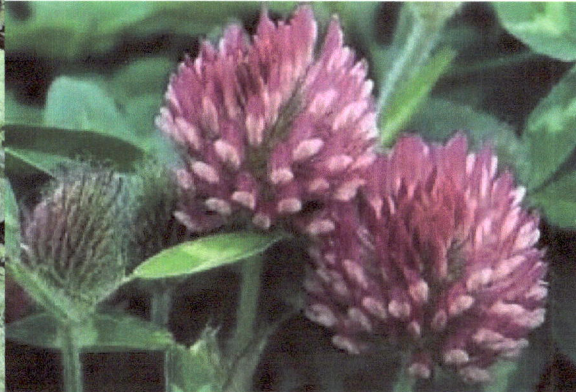
Red Clover

The flowers and roots can be made into syrup, coffee and detoxifying tonics. But we just kill them so that we can have a 'beautiful' lawn and poison the other nutrient rich 'weeds' in the yard (chickweed, which can empower the body against allergies; plantain weed, commonly used for diaper rashes or skin irritants; and red clover, a lymphatic system cleanser.)

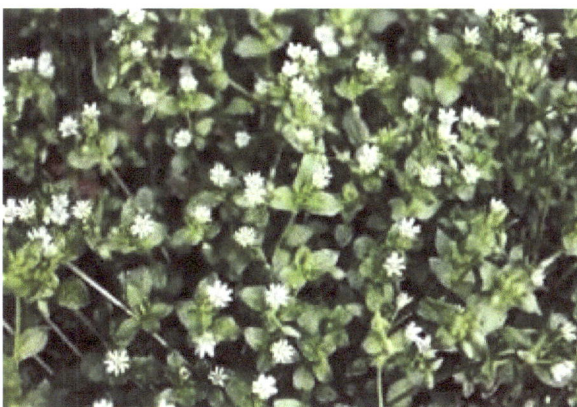
Chickweed

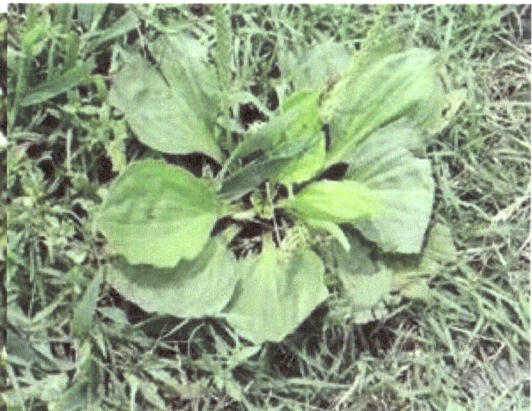
Plantain (wide leaf)

Sprinkle Chickweed and plantain weed in omelets, salads or just use as a tea. Dandelion leaves are great raw or cooked. Another naturally occurring beneficial weed is nettle. Nettle and Dandelion are off the chart with iron and potassium and are very cooling or alkaline for the body. Simply, they help digestion, stimulate circulation, balance the endocrine system and promote liver function. Eating these "super food" bitters can turn your health around. The sugar we inundate our bodies with these days are opposite to its need for bitters in the form of herbs, greens and roots. The further we are from this basic need the more acidic we make our bodies. Consequently, we develop diabetes, PMS, cancer, high blood pressure and a variety of now common medical conditions. Recent published studies state that changing your diet can stop the development of cancer. Several resources provide a template diet to begin on the anti-cancer path. However, few are as grass roots as the Workout Around My Day method.

In addition to bitters, we need colorful foods. These foods with natural occurring astaxanthin and other carotenoids give the body stamina, resistance in heat and build the immune system better than vitamin C and E. Astaxanthin is most readily available in salmon, which are known for their upstream struggle during spawning season. The astaxanthin gives them the stamina. This is the perfect example of "you are what you eat". In addition, an old health axiom tells us that carrots are good for our eyes. But more than just your eyes, other foods in this family like sweet potatoes and kale, can help your reproductive system function properly.

I have mentioned several recommendations here for small diet changes. In review:

- Eat in-season fruits and vegetables from the clean fifteen list or the organic versions of those on the dirty dozen list
- Shop at your local farmer's market or join a CSA
- Seek herbs and bitter greens to curb your sugar cravings
- Eat colorful foods

Below is an example of a simple recipe to try on your new path. It is also a pretty neat story on how to get your children on board. Enjoy! More recipes add the end of the book in the new Recipes section.

Detox Salad

So, one day I had a taste for something a little bit different. My children wanted beets and they were sitting in the kitchen waiting for me to crank out a meal. What could I do different with beets in a jiffy? "I want a salad but I want something warm and crunchy" I thought. So here it is!

3 medium carrots
4 beets
Wild spring mixed greens (dandelion, beet greens, lamb's quarters)
Arugula
Spinach
3 TBSP chia seeds
1 TBSP almonds or pistachios
1 TBSP coconut oil

2 inches of fresh minced ginger root
6-7 cloves of minced garlic
1 small onion minced

Serves 6

Coarsely cut carrots, beets and greens. Finely mince onions, ginger and garlic. Crunch the nuts. Over low heat warm oil and sauté onions and ginger. After two minutes, add garlic for about one minute. Sprinkle with vegetable curry seasoning (turmeric, cumin, coriander) and set aside. Meanwhile steam carrots and beets up to 15 minutes. Combine carrots and beets with the sauté mix. Spread arugula and wild mixed spring salad greens on a plate. Put two scoops of the carrot and beet mixture on top of greens, sprinkle with chia seeds and nuts. Sea salt to taste. No salad dressing required. Feel free to use the juice from the vegetable mix.

Root vegetables and bitter greens are best for digestion, bile secretion, liver cleansing or as we know it, detoxifying. Wild spring mixed salad greens can include dandelion, beet greens and spinach; not to mention the array of other vitamins and minerals therewith (A, B1-B12, C, D, E, K, Niacin, Biotin, Iron, Folate, etc.) Remember that the more bitter the greens, the higher they are in calcium, phosphorus, and magnesium. These are all bone and muscle building vitamins. The chia seeds and nuts, by the hand full, enhance these qualities and help to balance your sugar levels and add complete protein, making this salad a super antioxidant low calorie meal.

How to Make Every Bite Count

Society encourages us to graze. Even while we enjoy our favorite book or television show, we grab a bag of chips and munch. Most keep an action -packed schedule because our children *must* be "involved" in something. We are on the go so much, who has time to sit down and enjoy a meal with the family or even by ourselves. It is always grab and go from the nearest carry out or dare I say 'fast' food spot. Not the best way to inculcate good eating habits or nutrition. I separate the two because we end up modeling that food is a necessary evil, or a desire to satisfy. The choices are rarely nutritional. We even forget what nutrition is, and the real purpose of food. Food is a fuel for our body, mind and soul.

Society even pushes us into modes of fast and famine. When you finally have a minute to spend quality time with your family or friends and sit down to a good home cooked meal, it becomes an event. The great feast! We haven't enjoyed such companionship and deliciousness in so long that we overindulge. Then we feel guilty and go into famine mode. 'OMG look at how much I ate? I am going to have to starve myself all week to get back into my dress!'

How do we stop the grab and go mentality? How do we *not* graze? Does it always have to be feast or famine? Can it be feast with moderation? How do we learn to walk the middle path? The answer is to enjoy good wholesome food in the right time and balance it with hydration.

The key to making every bite count is to supply your body with the nutrition it needs on time. First thing in the morning your body has been working hard detoxifying and processing the food from yesterday. After so much work, it needs to be restored with good proteins. If you are in a rush, grab a quick bowl of Q'ia or oatmeal with in-season fruits, a room temperature glass of water or some herbal tea. Mid-morning give yourself a boost with a handful of nuts and dried fruits. (Here are some nut combinations below). Dried goji berries are considered a complete protein. Lunchtime go all out heavy on proteins balanced with raw fruits and vegetables. Seal off your meal with water or tea. That should hold you until six o'clock or dinnertime, whichever comes first. However, if you have a long commute or historically have an afternoon dip, make sure to have a Pro Bar handy.

Recommended combinations:

Almonds and dates – both are best known to stabilize sugar levels and high fiber content keeps you feeling full

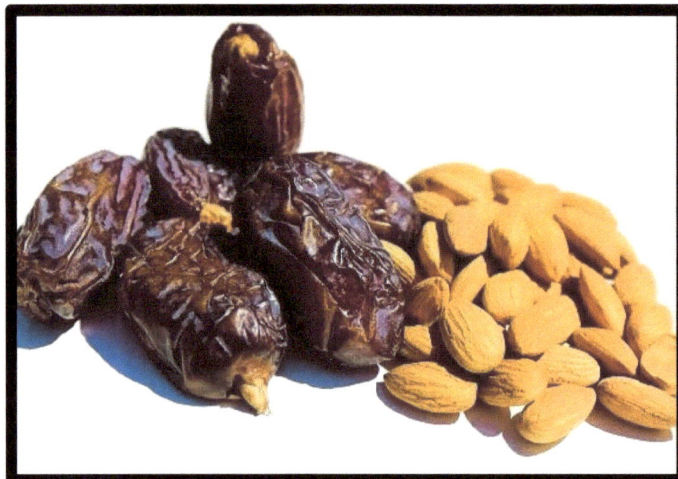

Golden berries and walnuts – Both have rarely vital phytonutrients that are anti-inflammatory and detoxify the body.

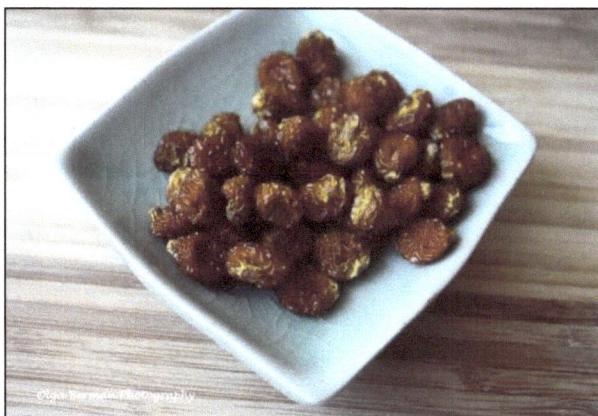

Goji berries and pistachios – Both known for highest nutrition value and can be considered a complete meal together.

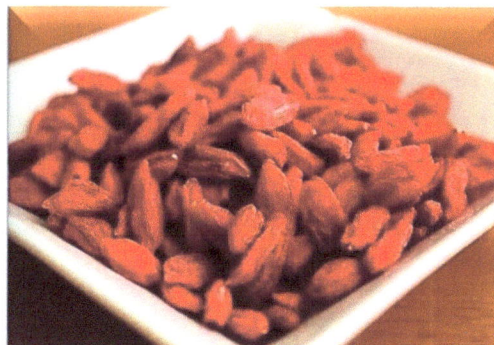

These will all make great choices for a perfect end to your day. Possibly, you may even choose them for a late afternoon pick me up.

More Powerful Food Choices

Now I am going to step back and give you some traditional views on food. Historically, some traditions prescribed (yes as in a medical prescription) certain foods for people based on their temperament. The four humors medicine model, which dates to ancient Egypt, was the basis of the Greco-Roman model used by Hippocrates. Other cultures continued to build on this in the East. During the Middle Ages in the 10th century, Avicenna in Persia wrote The Canon of Medicine. To this day, it is the most complete book detailing nutrition, treatments and other medical advice for doctors. It detailed how to balance temper of the variety of humors. He was the first to include emotional, mental, moral, self-awareness, movements and dreams.[4] The Canon of Medicine continued to be used until the eighteenth century. Western medicine rejected the theory around the turn of the nineteenth century. However, some of these ideas can still apply to eating habits and food choices and are currently used in the Waldorf teaching methods. The theory is that personality types are driven by the most prominent of the four bodily fluids (phlegm, blood, yellow bile and black bile). It further divides into hot/cold and dry/wet all the way to nine temperaments. They are sanguine (hot and wet, bitter), choleric (hot and dry, sweet), melancholic (cold and dry, sour) and phlegmatic (cold and wet, salty). Sanguine people are usually loquacious, carefree and pleasure-seeking people. Choleric people are egocentric and extroverted. Melancholic people are quiet and analytical introverts. Finally, the phlegmatic are private, patient and tolerant. Try to identify yourself with one of these types to help you understand which of the foods below can benefit you. For more information on the four temperaments, Wikipedia gives a good overview. I consult The Traditional Healer's Handbook by Hakim Chishti, which is largely based on The Canon of Medicine.

These are some of the common grocery store staples and things that we buy often. As you read, you will quickly see why expiration dates, reading labels and the condition of food are important.

Fruits:

Banana – hot in the first degree, has little use as a food, except for people with a very cold in temperament, who should eat it with honey.

Dried dates – should be eaten with almonds to annul any adverse effects.

Fig – fresh figs are preferred to dried. Although quite nourishing, they are very hot. It is a cure for piles and helps gout.

Olives and olive oil – the older olive oil is, the hotter it becomes. Olive oil is an excellent treatment for the skin and hair, and it delays old age.

Peach – generate cold, relax the stomach, and soften the bowels. A good laxative, they should be eaten before, rather than after a meal.

Spices

---

[4] Retrieved from Wikipedia, "Four Temperaments", origin of the citation is Lutz, Peter L. (2002). The Rise of Experimental Biology: An Illustrated History Humana Press. P. 60 IBSN 0896038351

Coriander Seed – alleviates flatulence and resolves fevers. It is an effective treatment of leukoderma, and it opens the subtlest networks of the veins. Excess moisture in the body is dried up by it, while milk flow, urine and menses are increased. It is great for colds, baldness, scalp problems and gray hair. The smoke of the burning seeds is an insect repellant.

Cinnamon – is hot in the third degree. Its volatile oil is great for indigestion.

Cumin – is very hot. It is the only spice or herb that travels through the stomach unaffected by digestion, until it reaches the liver. Soaked in water to create a tonic is great for colic.

Garlic – is hot in the third degree (meaning dry). It is used to dispel gas, promote menses, and expel afterbirth. It is excellent to correct cold in temperament, for dissolving phlegm, and the oil is used to treat insect bites.

Ginger- It is hot in the third degree and is best for softening phlegm. It also aids digestion.

Vinegar – is both cold and hot, nearly balanced between the two. Mixed with rose water, it is excellent for toothache and headache and alone dissolves phlegm.

Meats

Chicken – is light on the stomach and easy to digest. Considered hot and moist, it connects and balances all the essences, good for the brain and improves the complexion. However, overconsumption leads to gout. The best chicken is the one that has never laid an egg. We can only know the life of our food if we purchase from the farmer directly.

Other hot and moist meats include: lamb, veal, and shellfish.

Fish – Cool and moist. Fresh water fish is best, and those that feed on plant life, not mud or noxious gas. That means water that is not polluted. Salmon is an excellent source of omega-3 fatty acids, vitamin, immune-supportive selenium, muscle building protein, heart healthy niacin, vitamin B12, energy –producing phosphorus and heart healthy magnesium and vitamin B6.

Beef – Cool and dry not recommended as a daily food.

Mutton – Hot and dry not recommended as a daily food.

Legumes (for culinary purposes nuts are considered legumes)[5]

Lentils – All lentils produce dryness. Small amounts should be eaten, as a side dish. In larger quantities, it is generally bad for the stomach. However, some traditions say that it produces a sympathetic heart, tears in the eyes and removes pride.

Pistachios- It is said that eaten with egg yolk makes the heart strong. The reddish skin stems diarrhea and vomiting.

Rice –Next to wheat, it is the most nourishing grain. Tradition states that it increases pleasant dreams and semen.

Water – The best drink in this world and the next is water. Water is moist and because of this slightly cooling. It assists digestion of foods and absorption of nutrients. Eastern tradition says," When you are thirsty, drink [water] by sips ad do not gulp it down…Gulping water produces sickness of the liver."

You Can Work out Around Your Day

The previous chapter on food choices and diet addressed the largest factors in making powerful lifestyle changes. We have already nailed down 80% percent of the perspective shift in the program. The next step is to renew your view on movement. Here I will share with you my story on how exercise has changed my life and how it could change yours.

Until I had children, it never occurred to me that exercise was a necessity. I was no athlete by any stretch of the imagination. In fact, the thought of even going to the gym was ridiculous to me. Let me temper this and set the stage so you understand where I am coming from. I grew up in an era when you walked most places or took public transportation, a bus. Most often, my sister and I walked to the grocery store, which was about a mile away and each carried several pounds of groceries back home. My father took long morning walks with us, about four to six miles round-trip. When we returned, we stretch and did basic calisthenics to relax our muscles, then showered and had a high protein, full breakfast. It included turkey bacon, eggs with parsley and spices like cumin, whole wheat bread, grapefruit and grapes, sometimes pomegranate, tea and of course water. My father encouraged us by example to exercise often by doing push-ups and sit-ups, jumping jacks, etc. At the age of seventy, he managed to look about forty. He also taught us how to play tennis at his advanced age. In fact, exercise was such an integral part of my life that I accepted it like breathing.

---

[5] http://www.wisegeek.org/what-is-the-difference-between-a-nut-and-a-legume.htm

As an adult, I stopped walking and started driving long distances for work. Living in the suburbs, there are few sidewalks to walk long distances outside of the neighborhood. Only rarely are those sidewalks used and we often do not know our neighbors. You may have the occasional runner or dog walker. Then I had a child and another one. Despite being raised in a home where we had good wholesome food and had a balanced diet, I was not informed enough about nutrition specific to a woman's needs to prevent excess weight gain with my second pregnancy. During that time, I was also placed on bed rest complicating my weight control. For the first time in my life I was completely inactive! I had to find something to get me moving following my second pregnancy in a way that was not necessary the first time around. After investing in several DVDs, I eventually found what worked best for me; a combination of Pilates and weight training.

Strength training in general comes highly recommended from some of the top personal trainers today. I maintain my exercise routine twice a day once I reach my desired goal. Since I have the most energy earlier in the day, I use weights before breakfast to get my blood flowing and wake up to start my day. Just before dinner, I work more on Pilates and stretching type exercise. Most fitness workout articles I find are geared more towards men and are much longer than any workout I ever do. As a mother of six, I live by the mantra "less is more". When it comes to exercise that means 5 – 8 minutes' tops before the chaos starts. In fact, I find that a brief weight workout gives we the same feeling and vigor of a several- mile walk. Post workout I drink up to five glasses of water and eat a protein dense meal or snack followed by a calcium magnesium zinc supplement to feed my muscles. All within the comfort of my own home, I set a good example for my children and maintain my sanity.

From these beginning steps, especially after my second delivery, I have maintained a healthy weight, mental state and learned to better understand the things my father tried to implement in our diets and health habits. Recently I saw someone who I had not seen in ten years and they said that I had not changed. Embrace a routine of exercise in your daily life. It can stop the effects of aging while giving you a positive outlook on life.

Now let's talk about how we integrate several workouts into our daily routine.

Where are, we spending our time during the day?
- The bed
- The car
- The grocery store
- The office
- The playground
- The athletic field

Join me as we go through my day starting from the first moments of waking up. Still lying on my side in bed, I open my eyes. If I am on my right side, I start by doing hip-height leg lifts with my left leg, maintaining a flexed foot and then turning over and lifting the right leg as high as I can also with a flexed foot. Then I roll over onto my back, making sure to keep my tailbone straight as I gently lift my buttocks, holding each time five seconds longer than the time before. Now with my knees bent, I roll upright and scoot to the edge of my bed. Here I sit up alternately inhaling while pushing out my abs and exhaling while simultaneously pulling my abs towards my spine and sitting erect. Then I drop to my yoga mat on the floor by my bed and repeat the leg lift exercise on my left side. My next exercise is to flip onto my stomach and mimic swimming motion, moving opposite leg and arms. This is followed by moving into a body-plank and lifting my right leg eight times, keeping a pointed foot and switching to repeat with my left. Then it's time for five strong and deliberate push-ups. After these exercises, I roll up to a standing position and go to the bathroom. There I hold a five-pound weight in each hand as I squat, counting to 8 (the great 8) and holding the weights close to my waist. Then I stand holding the weights at my head's height and work my biceps. Then, holding the weights behind me, I continue to do squats, counting to 20 each time. Finally, I bend down and put the weights on the floor.

That's just getting out of bed. Now, I am fully energized and ready to start my morning.

Let's fast forward to the car. I drive distances that take usually between 35 minutes to an hour, often to run errands or take my kids to their activities. Usually I'm listening to music as I drive and I car-dance to the tunes. I would never recommend anything unsafe, and I encourage everyone to use their best judgment and skill. There are many surprising and completely safe ways to practice movement exercises while you are driving. What I am referring to are very small, intricate movements of the pelvis, thighs, hips, and core muscles. You have probably seen bellying dancing. Think of how slowly and detailed the hips must move.

You can try this now as you're reading. Sit on a chair and try to flex your buttocks. Now sit up straight and still flexing buttocks flex and move your knee muscles. Now get your thighs involved. What happens? Your hips automatically move. The catch is you must continue to sit up straight, which forces you to activate your core. Now make all those movements at once and flex your thighs and knees, while maintaining good posture, but do not use any force or pressure on your feet. This is car-dancing and doing a lower body workout. In fact, you can do the same seated at your desk, or anywhere. When you reach your destination, do a runner's stretch for each leg discretely by your car and move on.

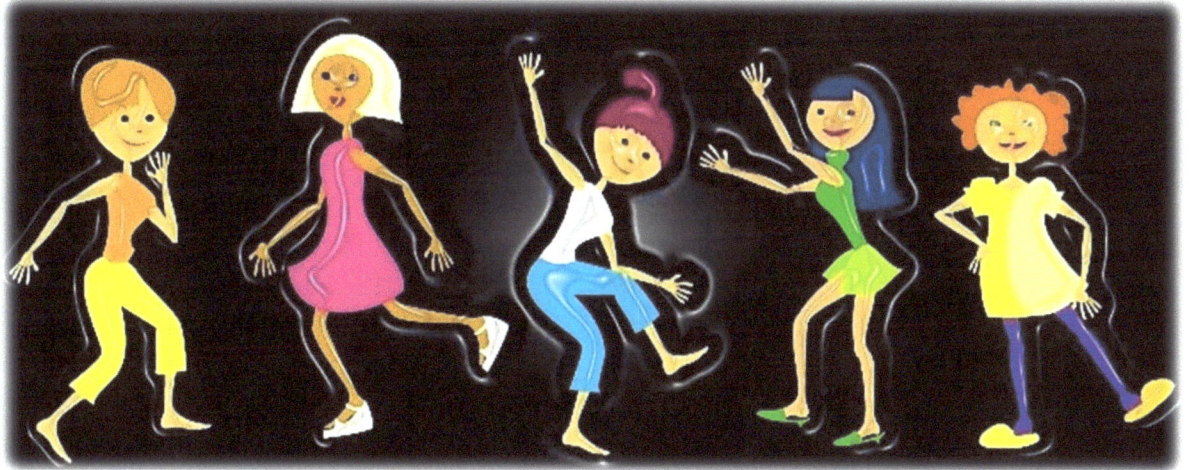

Normally walk or sit and read a book? I wrote most of my blog the other day at my son's soccer practice. I was standing and slowly and carefully kicking my legs forward yet still very close to my body, and then kicking backward. One at a time, I would alternate between small kicks forward, backward, and on either side. After a set of eight in each direction, I would quickly walk 100 yards. Then I stood in place again while typing on my iPhone. I do the same at the playground and most places outside.

If we stop and review – what part of my body am I constantly moving? It is my legs but with an emphasis on my thighs. Why? The thighs and legs are your powerhouse. Most women carry weight in their thighs. When this area is, strong and moving, you are energized. Conversely, when you are not moving they lose their muscle tone and weigh you down.

Of course, let us not overlook the oldie but goodies: Calisthenics. Jumping jacks, jumping rope, push-ups, crunches and squats. None of these takes more than five minutes to do and work all major muscle groups, burn more calories per pound (the heavier you are the more you burn) and are energizing and mind clearing. Take an extra five minutes for yourself and mix it up.

How to Make Every Movement Count

For most women. our lower half is the challenge zone. Our thighs and buttocks are the last to slim down. The reason for this is that upwards of 45% of our body weight is in our thighs. Beginning at puberty, when we need the extra fat, our "motherly zone" (breast, hips and thighs), start to accumulate an extra layer of fat in preparation for childbearing. Historically during this time cultures have introduced girls to movements or dance to strengthen that area. Sadly, as we have evolved, we have moved away from this traditional practice. Most of those movements were part of women's daily chores. For example, she would squat in the garden; walk with heavy baskets of harvest or water vases upraised; and stand while cooking. Any of these activities sound familiar? The dances would be ceremonial and in all female company because it involved intricate hip and thigh circulation. Does this maybe remind you of some modern day African or Latin dances? It goes without saying in our automated world, we do none of these daily activities and certainly are not taught any specific movements at puberty. I will focus on ways to avoid accumulation (or further accumulation) of fat cells, movements that you can incorporate daily, and how to keep it off.

First, whenever possible, stand instead of sitting. Sitting for long periods, i.e. working a desk job or daily watching TV for hours deactivates the muscles in your leg. That means you are creating an environment of muscle loss. Additionally, you are priming your muscles to permanently adhere to the fat cells floating between them.

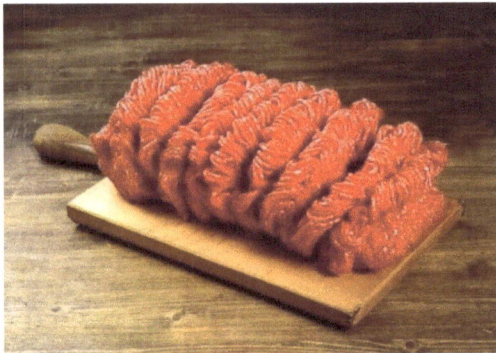

Your thighs without movement

Recent studies show that you can reverse the effects of inactivity by moving at least an hour per day. There are so many opportunities do this especially if you make it your habit to move ten minutes at the end of every hour. Most people are awake at least fourteen hours per day. That can easily add up to 140 minutes or over two hours of opportunities to incorporate movement. Many companies today are promoting a standing desk environment. Whether you work outside the home or stay home, you can work out around your day.

Cleaning is a great way to stay in shape. Here are some ideas:

- ❏ Do squats while picking things up from the floor
- ❏ Stand straight doing the breathing while sweeping
- ❏ Go up and down the stairs twisting at the waist sideways

Marching will get those thighs pumping ladies and stave off excess. Whenever possible and no one is looking just march for about 50 yards or 10 paces during your day.

Another thing we don't think about is our posture. Even while standing keeping your back straight works your core muscles. It does not seem to be movement but it is. Did you know that there are 35 muscle groups in the core? More than the muscles illustrated below, the hips, buttocks, and the thighs are also considered parts of the core.

Core stability muscles

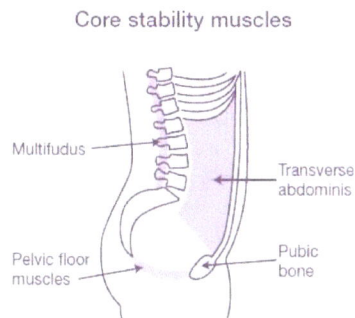

Multifudus
Transverse abdominis
Pelvic floor muscles
Pubic bone

Along with good posture comes best breathing practices; another thing we take for granted. Believe it or not, there is a right and a wrong way to breathe. Most of us, due to our posture are not breathing correctly. Here again practicing better breathing is excellent for digestion and energy boosting.

Walking is always the simplest option. You don't have to play sports, dance or even march; just take a walk.

In review, how can you work out throughout your day?

1. Stand more often

2. Enhance your daily activities like cleaning

   Do intermittent squatting: stay in a squat for thirty seconds
   Shift your weight from one leg to the other by lifting behind you
   Do standing tick tocks like a clock from side to side

3. March. There are more opportunities throughout your day to activate muscle burn.

   Starting your day with weight bearing lunges turns on your metabolism and tells it to burn fat

Use the stairs instead of the elevator or escalator whenever possible
End your day doing mountain climbers

4. Watch your posture
5. Breathe and take a walk

So, you see it's not hard to make every movement count. Just be more conscious of how and when you move. Remember the human body was meant to move. Make these new choices you have learned and adapted to meet your goal and establish healthy habits. Doesn't it feel better to fit into those jeans in the back of the closet? Well, why not keep wearing them? You will find over time you will not only have definition but have more energy… not to mention a spring in your step!

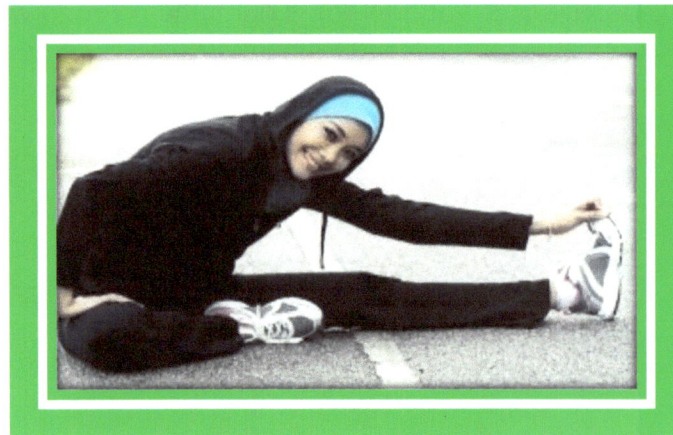

Workout Around My Day:

Top Ten on the Go Health Tips

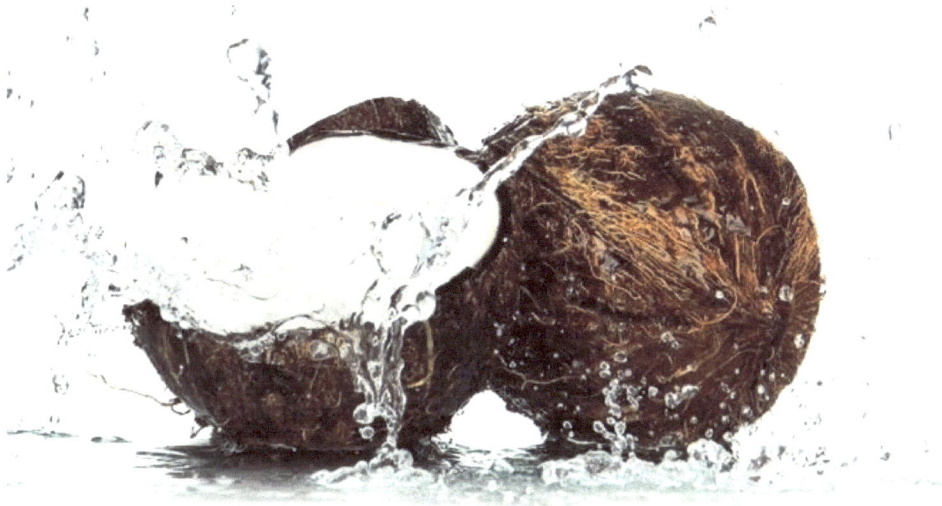

☐ Select hydrating foods and raw produce from the clean fifteen list

☐ Read your bread labels if you must when you eat it

☐ Learn to make your own bread

☐ Substitute dark greens for bread in sandwiches

☐ Substitute sweet potatoes or avocadoes for condiments in sandwiches

☐ Substitute sweet potatoes for rice when eating red meat

☐ Sprinkle dried herbs like nettle leaf or cilantro on meals salads or rice dishes

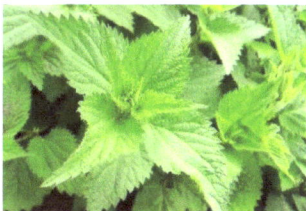

Nettle Leaf

☐ Snack on nuts or seeds

☐ Bring lots of water, or some coconut water and hydrating snacks

☐ Skip the sugary snacks (cookies, crackers, candy, chocolate, carbonated beverages, sweet tea, etc.)

Your Turn: Interactive Section

Exercise One: Reflect on How Eat

In the next few pages, let's see where you are now. To change you should know what you are doing that works well and what you are doing that does not. The only way to understand yourself better is to document and record your habits. This is the first step to becoming more mindful in eating, movement or anything.

Just like with the portion control challenge, notice whether you are satisfied or hungry after meals and snacks. Also, include as best you can the number of ounces that you are drinking and what you are drinking. Be honest if it is juice, a latte, a sweet tea or water. What you drink contributes to being satisfied or hungry. For example, I notice when I drink a latte on an empty stomach as a snack, I crash and burn. Whereas, if I have it after a full meal, I may fill satisfied and energetic. Everything going in your body makes a difference.

First record what goes in your mouth for the next five days, on the eating log. You can start now even if it is already evening. Record the time you eat and what you are eating. There are many apps for this or get a composition book for five days. Include your beverages with each meal and snack and mark whether you are satisfied or still hungry after eating.

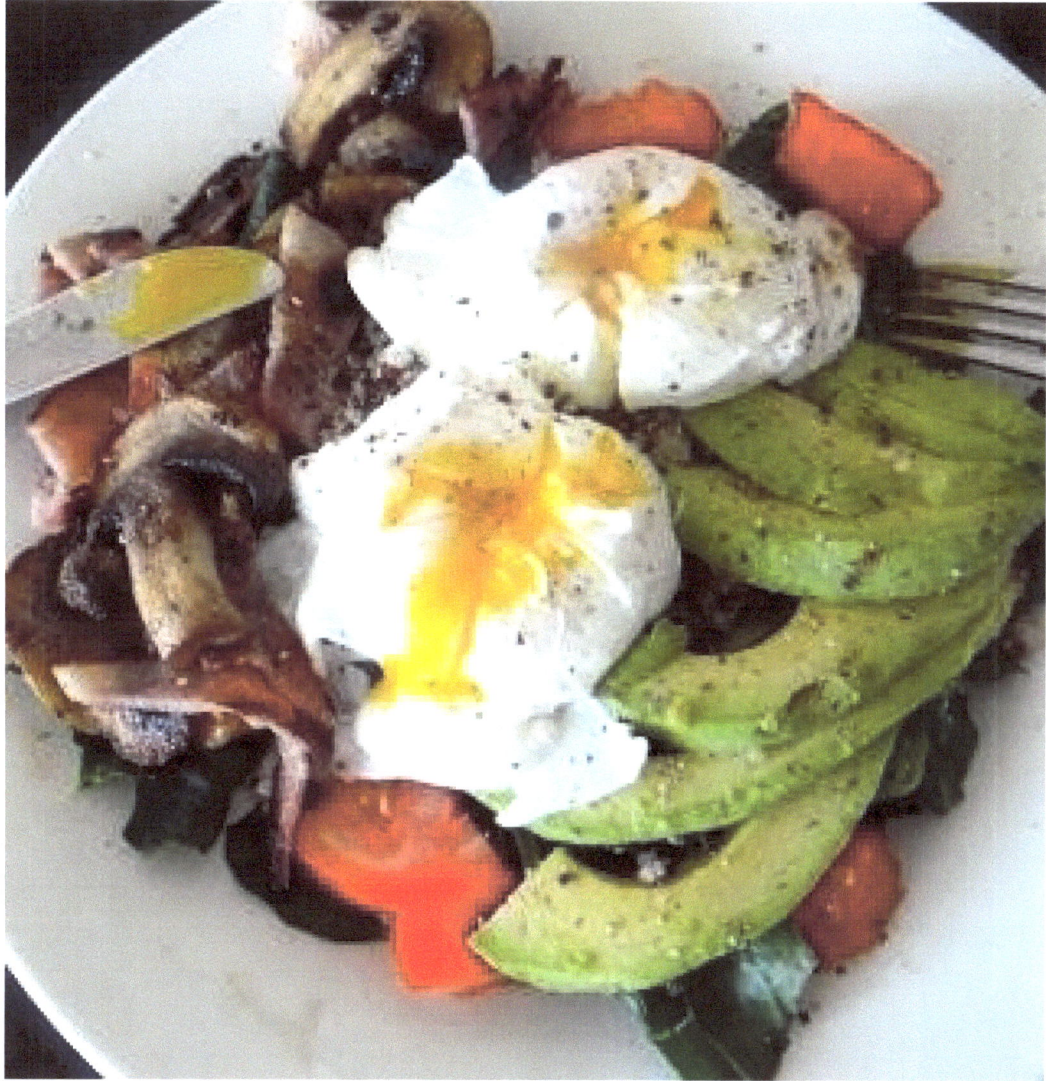

How am I eating? Is it healthy?

Today

_____
_____
_____
_____

Morning ___ Satisfied___ Hungry

_____
_____
_____
_____

Afternoon ___ Satisfied___ Hungry

_____
_____
_____
_____

Snack ___ Satisfied ___ Hungry

_____
_____
_____
_____

Evening ___ Satisfied___ Hungry

Day 2

_____
_____
_____
_____

Morning ___ Satisfied___ Hungry

_____
_____
_____
_____

Afternoon ___ Satisfied___ Hungry

_____
_____
_____
_____

Snack ___ Satisfied ___ Hungry

_____
_____
_____
_____

Evening ___ Satisfied___ Hungry

Day 3

_____
_____
_____
_____

Morning ___ Satisfied___ Hungry

_____
_____
_____
_____

Afternoon ___ Satisfied___ Hungry

_____
_____
_____
_____

Snack ___ Satisfied ___ Hungry

_____
_____
_____
_____

Evening ___ Satisfied___ Hungry

Day 4

_____
_____
_____
_____

Morning ___ Satisfied___ Hungry

_____
_____
_____
_____

Afternoon ___ Satisfied___ Hungry

_____
_____
_____
_____

Snack ___ Satisfied ___ Hungry

_____
_____
_____
_____

Evening ___ Satisfied___ Hungry

Day 5

_____
_____
_____
_____

Morning ___ Satisfied___ Hungry

_____
_____
_____
_____

Afternoon ___ Satisfied___ Hungry

_____
_____
_____
_____

Snack ___ Satisfied ___ Hungry

_____
_____
_____
_____

Evening ___ Satisfied___ Hungry

Exercise Two: Look for opportunities for improvement

Now that you will see how you are eating, what you are eating, when you are eating and the result. Review your food journal after 3 – 5 days. Let's see how we can improve. What to look for:

Skipped meals

Regular snacking

Rarely drinking water

Times you are eating and drinking

Are you still hungry after eating?

If not, what did you eat? What time of day is it?

If so, what did you eat? What time of day is it?

These are areas that need improvement.

Exercise Three: Are You Dehydrated?

Did you know that sometimes when we eat we are truly thirsty? Reach for a glass of water before you reach for food and see if you are full.

Exercise Four: Start Your Day with Breakfast

Retrain your body with nourishment. Below are some sample breakfast meals to try. Flip to the bonus section for recipes.

- Oatmeal with in season fruits or dates, coconut oil or walnut oil
- Boiled eggs, salad, real whole grass fed milk cheese or goat chevre, in season fruit
- Beverages: water, herbal tea, black coffee or espresso
- Energizing smoothie, plant protein rich smoothie

Today

_____
_____
_____
_____

Morning ___ Satisfied___ Hungry

_____
_____
_____
_____

Afternoon ___ Satisfied___ Hungry

_____
_____
_____
_____

Snack ___ Satisfied ___ Hungry

_____
_____
_____
_____

Evening ___ Satisfied___ Hungry

Day 2

_____
_____
_____
_____

Morning ___ Satisfied___ Hungry

_____
_____
_____
_____

Afternoon ___ Satisfied___ Hungry

_____
_____
_____
_____

Snack ___ Satisfied ___ Hungry

_____
_____
_____
_____

Evening ___ Satisfied___ Hungry

Day 3

_____
_____
_____
_____

Morning ___ Satisfied___ Hungry

_____
_____
_____
_____

Afternoon ___ Satisfied___ Hungry

_____
_____
_____
_____

Snack ___ Satisfied ___ Hungry

_____
_____
_____
_____

Evening ___ Satisfied___ Hungry

Day 4

_____
_____
_____
_____

Morning ___ Satisfied___ Hungry

_____
_____
_____
_____

Afternoon ___ Satisfied___ Hungry

_____
_____
_____
_____

Snack ___ Satisfied ___ Hungry

_____
_____
_____
_____

Evening ___ Satisfied___ Hungry

Day 5

_____
_____
_____
_____

Morning ___ Satisfied___ Hungry

_____
_____
_____
_____

Afternoon ___ Satisfied___ Hungry

_____
_____
_____
_____

Snack ___ Satisfied ___ Hungry

_____
_____
_____
_____

Evening ___ Satisfied___ Hungry

Now that you have taken these few days to review, reflect, compare, contrast how you feel with your new food choices and eating times as compared to the previous five days.

Are you remembering to use your new food choices? Did you skip any meals? How did it make you feel?

Are you often dehydrated? If so, does it make you eat more? What are your choices your new go to foods?

Exercise Five: A Movement Reflection

In the next few pages, look at where you are now. For the first day record your movement and exercise as you are. How many hours are you sitting? How many hours are you commuting? Do you sit up straight or do you have good posture?

Starting from Day 2 try adding ten minutes of movement per waking hour (stairs, pacing, marching, jumping jacks, etc.)

Starting from Day 3 dedicate at least two of ten- minute slots to a specific workout like the examples above (jumping jacks, push- ups, squats, marching, etc.) Also, try using a standing desk at work or balance ball to help with your posture. Add a ten-minute workout each day until to have five that you can maintain. Record movement for five days.

Examples

Today	Day 2	Day 3	Day 4	Day 5
Slouching at breakfast			Good posture at breakfast	
One-hour commute sitting	One-hour commute sitting	One-hour commute sitting	One-hour commute sitting	One-hour commute sitting
Ankle circles at desk			Stability ball while sitting	
Sat for 2 hours in meeting				
	Squats while cleaning	Walked at soccer practice		Walked at track practice

Your Turn! Record Your Daily Movements

Today

_____
_____
_____
_____

Morning ___Tired___ Energetic ___ No Change

_____
_____
_____
_____

Afternoon ___Tired___ Energetic ___ No Change

_____
_____
_____
_____

Evening ___ Tired ___ Energetic___ No Change

Your Turn! Record Your Daily Movements

Day 2 – Dedicate two ten-minute slots to jumping jacks, push- ups, squats, or stairs.

_____
_____
_____
_____

Morning ___Tired___ Energetic ___ No Change

_____
_____
_____
_____

Afternoon ___Tired___ Energetic ___ No Change

_____
_____
_____
_____

Evening ___ Tired ___ Energetic___ No Change

Your Turn! Record Your Daily Movements

Day 3 – Dedicate two ten-minute slots to jumping jacks, push- ups, squats, or stairs.

_____
_____
_____
_____

Morning ___Tired___ Energetic ___ No Change

_____
_____
_____
_____

Afternoon ___Tired___ Energetic ___ No Change

_____
_____
_____
_____

Evening ___ Tired ___ Energetic___ No Change

Your Turn! Record Your Daily Movements

Day 4 – Dedicate three ten-minute slots to jumping jacks, push- ups, squats, or stairs.

_____
_____
_____
_____

Morning ___Tired___ Energetic ___ No Change

_____
_____
_____
_____

Afternoon ___Tired___ Energetic ___ No Change

_____
_____
_____
_____

Evening ___ Tired ___ Energetic___ No Change

Your Turn! Record Your Daily Movements

Day 5 – Dedicate four ten-minute slots to jumping jacks, push- ups, squats, or stairs.

_____
_____
_____
_____

Morning ___Tired___ Energetic ___ No Change

_____
_____
_____
_____

Afternoon ___Tired___ Energetic ___ No Change

_____
_____
_____
_____

Evening ___ Tired ___ Energetic___ No Change

Being Consistent with the Workout

Use the following daily calendar to access your daily schedule. If you have extraordinarily busy day, use one for that. There are two sets of three; one for each weekday sample days (The Normal Day and The Crazy Day), and one for the weekend. I am calling them: The Normal Day, The Crazy Day and The Weekend Day.

On the first set, document your time as you currently live. I will give further instructions on how to use the second set afterwards. Although this broken into 30 minute intervals split them into 15 - minute sections. Remember the goal here is to find up to 15 minutes where you can steal away to exercise.

So, what to look for? The times that you are on social media - yes that counts- FB, Twitter, Instagram, Google chat, whatever. Give it another place in your schedule, maybe at the end of week. (Screen time at the end of the day interrupts your ability to sleep.) Document and times of these activities and trade that time for a better choice, your health! Other windows of opportunity are times that you are sitting and watching TV or playing Mind Craft or other video games or chatting on the phone. The times that you are snacking…lol, caught ya! You get the idea.

Here is the best part! You have learned how to change and integrate new eating habits and movement habits. Now let's get into fitting actual workouts in your crazy schedule.

Once you document each day type, start looking for those 10-minute opportunities to exercise.

Repeat this process with your weekend sheets. First document throughout your day, looking for the 10-minute windows. Then re-create your schedule with the second set of sheets.

Happy scheduling!

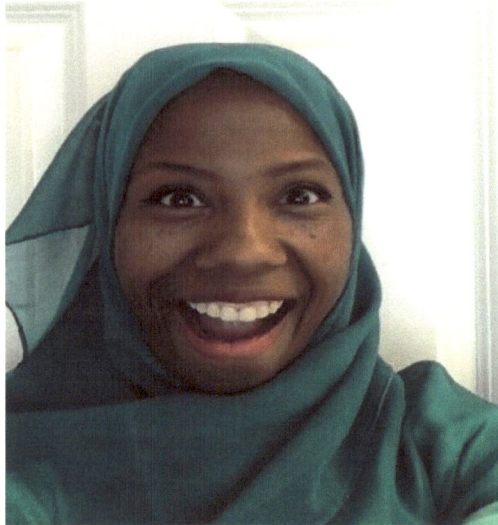

See my example below.

Time	Appointment	To Do
7:00 AM	Wake up; exercise routine	Put on dinner during breakfast
7:15 AM	shower; dress	meat in pressure cooker
7:30 AM	make protein shake or oatmeal and cook breakfast	brown rice in vita clay cooker
7:45 AM	sit down eat egg frittata with fresh fruits and drink water with kids	chop up salad mix and place in frig
8:00 AM	Prep to leave the house and pack everyone into the car	
8:15 AM	drive; drop; commute	
9:00 AM	Arrive at work	

Time	Appointment	Errands
12:00 PM	Lunch Break; climb stairs before lunch	
12:15 PM	eat lunch	pick up kids
1:00PM	return to office	soccer practice
3:00PM	Mid- afternoon stretch/ march	

Time	Appointment	
5:00PM	leave office for pick ups	
6:00PM	Soccer practice/walk or other exercise	
7:30PM	return home; rejuvenation workout	
7:45PM	shower; set dinner out from Vitaclay pot or pressure cooker	
8:15 PM	dinner time clean up	**Calls**
8:30 PM	Bed time routine starts	
9:00PM	Lights out; stretch work out and Me-time for you	
9:15 PM	water and sleep	

Starting today record your actual weekday schedule.

Time	Appointment	To Do
7:00 AM		
7:15 AM		
7:30 AM		
7:45 AM		
8:00 AM		
8:15 AM		
9:00 AM		
12:00 PM		**Errands**
12:15 PM		
1:00PM		

Time	Appointment	
3:00PM		
5:00PM		
6:00PM		
7:30PM		
7:45PM		
8:15 PM		**Calls**
8:30 PM		
9:00PM		
9:15 PM		

Record your weekend schedule.

Time	Appointment	To Do
7:00 AM		
7:15 AM		
7:30 AM		
7:45 AM		
8:00 AM		
8:15 AM		
9:00 AM		
12:00 PM		**Errands**
12:15 PM		

Time	Appointment		
1:00PM			
3:00PM			
5:00PM			
6:00PM			
7:30PM			
7:45PM			
8:15 PM		**Calls**	
8:30 PM			
9:00PM			
9:15 PM			

Starting today record your actual crazy day schedule.

Time	Appointment	To Do	
7:00 AM			
7:15 AM			
7:30 AM			
7:45 AM			
8:00 AM			
8:15 AM			
9:00 AM			
12:00 PM		**Errands**	

Time	
12:15 PM	
1:00PM	
3:00PM	
5:00PM	
6:00PM	
7:30PM	
7:45PM	
8:15 PM	**Calls**
8:30 PM	
9:00PM	
9:15 PM	

Make New Schedule with workouts included with the next set of sheets.

Time	Appointment	To Do
7:00 AM		
7:15 AM		
7:30 AM		
7:45 AM		
8:00 AM		
8:15 AM		
9:00 AM		

Time		Errands
12:00 PM		
12:15 PM		
1:00PM		
3:00PM		
5:00PM		
6:00PM		
7:30PM		
7:45PM		
8:15 PM		Calls
8:30 PM		
9:00PM		
9:15 PM		

Weekend Day

Time	Appointment	To Do
7:00 AM		
7:15 AM		
7:30 AM		
7:45 AM		
8:00 AM		
8:15 AM		

Time		Errands
9:00 AM		
12:00 PM		
12:15 PM		
1:00PM		
3:00PM		
5:00PM		
6:00PM		
7:30PM		
7:45PM		
8:15 PM		**Calls**
8:30 PM		
9:00PM		
9:15 PM		

Crazy Day

Time	Appointment	To Do
7:00 AM		
7:15 AM		
7:30 AM		
7:45 AM		
8:00 AM		

8:15 AM	
9:00 AM	
12:00 PM	**Errands**
12:15 PM	
1:00PM	
3:00PM	
5:00PM	
6:00PM	
7:30PM	
7:45PM	
8:15 PM	**Calls**
8:30 PM	
9:00PM	
9:15 PM	

Make self-nurturing a practice everyday

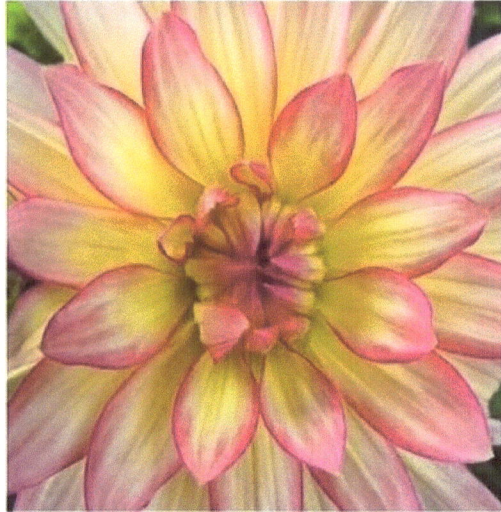

Not Just on Spa Day

WWW.WORKOUTAROUNDMYDAY.COM

How does it feel to re-create your time to include you as a priority? Was it a challenge for you to commit to the documenting or scheduling piece? What were those challenges? Did you forget the book? Did you let something or someone come between you are your choice?

The next section with address the mindset in making our choices. This is what I call the rest of the story or the **self-nurturing** piece of our well-being.

Ready for a lifestyle upgrade? Changing your choices, the way you eat and the way you move are only the beginning. The mindset and self-nurturing piece is what makes it a lifestyle change. You loving you, cherishing you and knowing that your physical and mental needs take precedence is the foundation of total well-bring.

The Rest of the Story

To be successful with the program, start making goals. Goals are the key to success with any program but especially this one. You need to find a way to work up to 5 workouts per day. Goal setting is important to see where you need to act. Then be committed to yourself.

In review, here is the Workout Around My Day™ Method:

- Document your habits and reflect
- Restructure your mindset and daily schedule
- Train yourself to make better choices
- Re-create your choices and daily schedule to include them

Get a simple folder (like a report cover or a binder) and print the daily logs and journals. Start jotting down what you put in your mouth for five days. Replace unhealthy choices with the recommended choices. Create your new meal plan and shopping list with those choices. Repeat this process with your movement. Then finally properly exercise. Learn how to make better choices for your new life. You will be stronger, live longer and live well.

In the first half of this book, I have tried to share with you how I have used this method as both a working mom and a stay at home mom. Using examples and strategies that have worked for some of my clients, I have made the implementation process seamless. One thing that each client has realized is the power of her mind. Believe me it does not get easier; you just learn how to embrace more. What makes this so important is that as mothers we rarely have a period of separation from our jobs, our children or our husbands for ourselves. Even if you have the best in-laws, babysitter or work/life balance job, you owe it to yourself to take time for yourself. There is more to staying healthy than just moving and eating better. You need to believe that you are worth it. I am talking about **mind set** and **self-nurturing**. Here are some basic steps to start a self-nurturing practice. I go into greater detail on understanding and recognizing your triggers in my online course Take Care of You. (For more details go to workoutaroundmyday.com.)

Building a Self-Nurturing System

- **Smile at yourself** in the mirror first thing in the morning even before washing your face. Then again afterward. Smiling is the best compliment you can pay yourself. It will brighten your own day and help you practice reflecting that to others all day long
- **Before breakfast**, shower and dressing take an extra 2-3 minutes to do a fitness challenge. (Squats, jump rope, plank, walking plank, challenge yourself physically for 2-3 minutes and put on the timer on your phone.)
- **Take an extra 1-2 minutes** to look at yourself after dressing, putting on make- up (if you wear make- up) doing your hair and put those finishing touches as if you are going somewhere special. Feeling good about the way you look goes a long way.
- **Make yourself breakfast**. A good balanced breakfast complete with a glass of water, a fresh fruit, some seeds or nuts or other source of protein and fat, and a fresh vegetable.
- **Take one more minute** to meditate, pray or focus on positive self-talk to start your day.

These are the very basic tenants of loving you. We throw around this word self-care so much that we don't even understand the meaning.

The actual definition is:

Providing proper nutrition, sleep, physical movement, medical preventative care and a stress reducing activity to maintain total well-being.

"It's all about falling in love with yourself and sharing that love with someone who appreciates you, rather than looking for love to compensate for a self- love deficit" -Eartha Kitt

---

Renewing Your Perspective

Making a lifestyle change is renewing your perspective. Whatever your challenge, food, exercise, time management, be the shift in your life. Dr. Mary Hemphill in her January 24, 2015 article called "Perspective Shifting", 'Being negative toward people & situations, annihilates any opportunity to shift your position or perspective. In fact, my colleague shared that **"being negative is**

perhaps the lowest form of existence."' Whoa! That hits home for me. Negative self- talk is the lowest form of thought. How do you elevate your mind…Free your mind!

Reflect on this for a minute. For example, if you tell yourself, 'I will never have the time to cook healthy food'; you will manifest it in your life through your actions. When you go to the grocery store, you will not seek the produce department or the sections in the store with healthier choices. So, start by telling yourself, I can cook healthy meals. Next seek assistance. You have already taken that step by purchasing and reading this book. Get an accountability partner or join one of the personalized coaching **programs**. Or a minimum seek for help in the grocery store. Now that you have reflected on ways to make a mind shift, commit to it!

Commit to reaffirming your new mindset. Reflection is the first step in this process. Make it happen by your commitment. Commitment comes in the form of reaffirming your positive thoughts whenever a negative thought creeps in. Here comes the negative thought: 'I did not sleep well last night, so no workout today". The overshadowing commitment says,' I will do it for at least ten minutes today'. Most of the workouts in my programs are ten minutes or less.

Act on your positive choices. Great! You have overcome hurdle number one with your mindset and commitment. Act! Have your yoga mat or blanket or towel next to your bed before you sleep at night and get on the floor first thing every morning. Make it happen! You think you can. You know you can. You can.

Rinse and repeat.

> *"My recipe for life is not being afraid of myself, afraid of what I think or of my opinions."- Eartha Kitt*

Setting a Foundation:

You have made it to a new beginning. **The steps for renewing your perspective are:**

1. **Reflect**
2. **Commit**
3. **Act**
4. **Rinse and repeat**

Now set the foundation for that perspective to make it actionable.

Just like building a structure you must have a foundation. In an architecture class that my children took, they experimented with columns, pillars, circles and squares. The most solid and stronger foundation had smaller, thicker and shorter pillars. As the structure gets taller, the pillars are thinner, taller and fewer. So, drawing from this as an analogy, build a foundation with small, deliberate, meaningful steps. As you walk your new path, it will become easier. You will get to a point when you can walk the path in longer less deliberate steps and bear more weight.

For example, at one point I changed my website from a template based website to a Word press website. I was very hesitant on this new path because Word press is all 'widgets' and 'plugins' oh my! But I was determined to build something to my specifications unhindered by a restricting template. I watched some tutorials and read about the process on the Word press forum and in less than 24 hours, I moved all my content over and switched my domain. Furthermore, within a week, I had worked out all of kinks and even created a pop up and squeeze page. Kept moving forward with the maintenance of posting my articles, and sending out my newsletter.

Start with a vision. Do the research and take a leap of faith. Make things happen. You are your own worst enemy. I could have held myself back with the fear of 'widgets' and 'plugins'. Months ago, that is exactly what drove me to a template based web site. But the overwhelming inconvenience of not being able to present the information that I wanted to, the way I wanted to propelled me to make an overdue change.

Applying this to your own health journey, is it better to stick with eating, sleeping and doing the things that are easy? Or is the overwhelm of the results of poor food, sleep and exercises choices propelling you to make an overdue change? Will it take a severe diagnosis from your doctor to encourage you commit to nurturing yourself? Is it better to invest in health insurance rather than making healthy choices with every movement and bite? Set the foundation of making yourself a priority by applying the exercises you use in this book to build your self-nurturing program. Start in this moment and try something new. It will take a mindset shift.

Mindset

OUR LIFE IS THE

SUM TOTAL OF ALL

THE DECISIONS WE

MAKE EVERY DAY,

AND THOSE DECISIONS ARE

DETERMINED BY OUR PRIORITIES.

-MYLES MONROE-

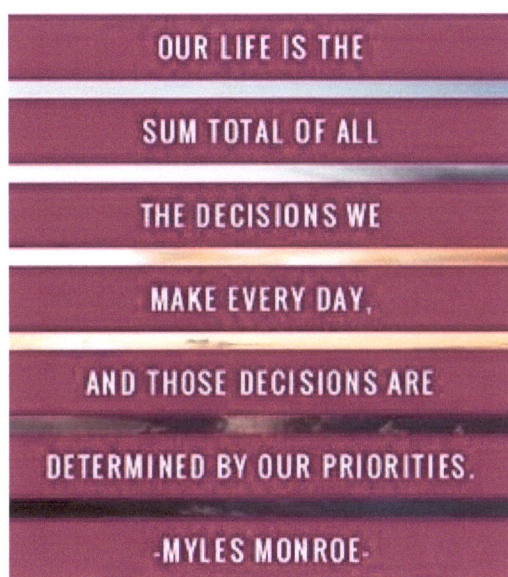

We often hear about having an attitude of gratitude. What does that mean and how do you get there? Does it have to do with our decisions? What are our triggers for our decisions? Our priorities determine or choices in the moment. We need make choice that are sustainable. So, the first building block to your new perspective and foundation is a sustainable pattern of behaviors. That means be grateful for the small things. Sometimes it just means being forgiving with yourself.

For example, if you miss sleep. It does not do a body good to exercise without all the other necessary components – sleep, food, energy. The mind is in survival mode compensating for the lack of sleep. In that state, you cannot override it and be all or nothing with your workout. At the same time, you must pay close attention to your nutrition when you miss sleep because coffee and foods with slowing sugars will send your adrenal system stir-crazy. A simple bowl of oatmeal with ½ tablespoon of coconut oil and a banana is best to jump start your body in the right direction followed by a cup of room temperature water. No brain fog, enough protein and proper sugars. Make the choices to do something great nutritionally for your body to compensate for lack of sleep so that you will have the energy to start your day and plan for an abbreviated workout midday.

- **Be clear on your goal. Make a meal plan based on your intention.** Remember 80% of health is tied to nutrition. There are thousands of discoveries, rediscoveries and announcements about the latest super food, 'belly fat zapping food', etc. everyday. So, where do you start? Only buy whole foods and not the processed versions of them, like oranges instead if orange juice. In earlier chapters, we have gone into detail on the building blocks of how to make a meal plan.

- **Positive self-talk. Be kind and gentle with yourself**. You cannot go from little or no activity to a full on HIIT daily workout. However, you can build a sustainable stabilization workout ten minutes a few times a day. Over the course of a month you could build up your stamina to graduate to a HIIT workout. Having an accountability partner or coach can help with your self-talk. In our weekly or bi-weekly check-in calls, when you are enrolled in a Workout Around My Day program, we will reinforce your positive self-talk and strengthen your perspective.

- **Action items. Just do it!** Seeing the results of your plan will keep you on track. Walking the path is better than just knowing the path. The more you walk the stronger your belief becomes. The stronger your belief the firmer your mindset. Make the plan, tell yourself you can do it and get it done!

- It is easier than we make it. You can make it happen so just do it!

Commit

> *"Start where you are.*
> *Use what you have.*
> *Do what you can."*
>
> *Arthur Ashe*

It started snowing one afternoon and piled up to the door knob. I wanted to do a periscope demonstrating proper shoveling technique. Guess what? It was still snowing! I tried to do a scope with one hand and no shovel. In the end, I decided to do a periscope on post shoveling stretching. By the time my children woke up and I had a possible camera crew, there were other barriers. Sometimes life does not cooperate, it makes it hard to commit. But alas the snow ended on the next day and someone was willing and available to film. Then we had so much fun I forgot about it. But in a commitment to my audience, I offered a Live Q&A periscope instead. The challenges did not fit into the plan, right? We must learn how to make obstacles into opportunities. Here is my formula to help me stay committed no matter what.

Make a contingency plan. In this instance, I did not have one. In a controllable situation, not a blizzard or impromptu snow play, I would have a plan B available to execute. Here I had to just go with the flow. It is always best to have a contingency plan. For example, if your commitment is to exercise but you need to shovel, make the shoveling and walking in the snow your workout.

Improvise. In the case of natural disasters and situations beyond our control, you must be open to improvising. Sometimes life just leads you in a completely different direction. Look at the possibilities in your situation not the impossibilities.

In my periscope example, in the end I had to improvise. Flexibility is a key and healthy part of improvising. I was so focused on showing people how to shovel that it escaped my mind to show the importance of stretching afterwards. By not having the needed resources available, I could improvise and keep trying to provide value. I could not film the demonstration so I played with my children and chose another topic.

Keep trying. No matter the situation keep trying. Challenges are the perfect opportunity to evolve and grow as a person. I call them character building exercises. I can recall intending to get through a to do list of ten items. By the end of the day, I had only completed three. I was watching the clock which forced me to prioritize what was urgent and important over everything else on the list. The other items were also important just not urgent. I did what was best and I kept trying to do more. I completed the list the next day by noon.

Embrace Imperfection. We plan and life opens other avenues for us. Sometimes we must embrace that the plan was not meant to be for us. Life can be imperfectly perfect. I often see that what unfolds is better than anything I could have planned. It leaves me saying, 'Why didn't I think of that?" Remember having an attitude of gratitude minor readjustment. Recently, I had a speaking engagement and had prepared an elaborate talk. In the end, I had a more intimate audience than expected and spoke from heart instead of my notes. Beautiful how life brings us closer to our goals in a warmer way than we could imagine. I could have viewed it as less exposure or a waste of a great presentation. But it was so easy to see that it was what we all needed.

In review, take life in stride and relax. Commitment does not mean being strict or rigid. It just means that you complete the task, process, or accomplish goals. Use this formula:

1. Make a contingency plan
2. Improvise when needed
3. Keep trying
4. Embrace imperfection

Do your goals include becoming a better you? Check out my new course 7 Weeks to A Better You! Gradually over a period of seven weeks, I will show you recipes, movements, scheduling and core strengthening exercises to help you achieve your goal. You will commit and be successful!

> ## "If your ship doesn't come in, swim out to meet it!"
>
> ## Jonathan Winters
>
> WWW.WORKOUTAROUNDMYDAY.COM

Investing in Your health

Ever buy exercise equipment, workout DVD set or a gym membership? Did it sit in your closet or on your dresser for three weeks unused? How many times have you made it to the gym this week? Congratulations on taking that first step to investing in your health! Let me help you with follow through and implementation. You know that you are worth it. Follow this simple four step process to celebrate you!

- **Start by dissecting your schedule**. If you do not document your time, this is the time to start. Open Excel or Google Calendar and fill in your major commitments (work, doctor's appointments, family obligations, etc.) Now fill in your soft commitments. These are the things that are flexible or can be delegated like meal preparation, practice pick-ups, grocery shopping, etc. Finally block off the time that you sleep. Do you have any alone pockets of 15 minutes to an hour? For the shorter pockets of alone time try out that workout DVD set or get on your new exercise equipment. For the hour slots, go to the gym.

- **Next commit to times that you find**. Surprise, surprise! Now you have found the time. Commit to that time fill it in on your schedule. Aim for at least once a day for fifteen minutes. This is a mindset exercise. Make sure that you can make it happen.
- **Now plan to make it happen.** You are committed it is black and white on your schedule like everything else that has priority in your life. Will you need to find child care arrangements for the time you have committed? Negotiate with a friend, your spouse, your relative or do it during a nap   time or homework time for your child. Find a way to make it happen.
- **Execute, just do it! You are all set!** Pop in that DVD, hop on the elliptical or head to the gym. Try it once and you will enjoy it so much. Following through with your commitment, plan for yourself will make you real make you feel accomplished. Your body will thank you and so will you heart!
- **You are on your way to better health**! If you need more accountability than your spreadsheet or Google Calendar, seek a sustainable program like the Life Quality Changer.

Plan

Congratulations you are doing it! Keep it up. Until it is you. It takes a good actionable plan. Without it you will gear up for two weeks and then stop. Here are the steps to create a system for a plan that keeps giving.

Set goals with due date. When you set goals, give them a deadline. Goals without deadlines are dreams. For example, I do a radio show every Wednesday. I must have the first draft for my talking points completed by the previous Thursday and the final by Saturday morning. Sunday night, I am revising and integrating any additional research. I do one final review on Tuesday night and place it in my **action box** for Wednesday before going to sleep.

Schedule the baby steps. As you can see in my previous example, my baby steps have deadlines over a period of days. Step one is due within 24 hours of my last radio show. Step two is due two days later. Step three/ final step the night before. Step four my final product has an **action box.**

Enlist an accountability partner. I also have an accountability partner to light a fire under me…my listeners! I know that my audience is awaiting great content and I do not want to show up half-hearted. For you, it could a good friend, mentor, advisor, or partner. Someone who knows your due dates and deadlines and ping you with reminders.

Reward yourself. Once you achieve your goal reward yourself. Every week when I meet my goals, I reward myself by setting the bar higher. A reward does not always have to be tangible it could be just knowing that you are capable. Knowing that you are capable is have the battle of achievement! Now that you know you can do this, it is possible for you to achieve that! Keep setting your bar higher.

Rinse and repeat. And since you have done it once, you can do it twice. Keep up the great work. It is only the beginning of the amazing things to come.

Execute

Just make it happen! You have done your due diligence. Your head is in the game. For the past fifteen years, I have been perfecting, planning, honing, committing and implementing. I had been practicing different exercises, creating new recipes, and trying out new techniques. I had already committed to implementing and embracing a healthy lifestyle for myself and family. Nothing stark or drastic or too complicated. Something that I could enjoy and maintain. Daily I executed with every movement choice, grocery store list, cooking technique. When friends asked, 'what are you doing, you look great?' I concisely recounted as much detail as I could. Then someone said, 'I haven't seen you in ten years and you look the same. You should write a book.' One day, I decided to make it happen. I began to plan, commit and execute writing a book to share my methods with the world.

The plan was not to overwhelm but to invite. To give a little dose of the whole package. As you read my book, you will see my story unfold. My fitness and nutrition journey was gradual played out in so many different stages in my life. How would I capture those moments and make them relevant and relatable to my readers? As my plan evolved, I began to reach out for editors in my community to help me better shape and develop my story. Now with others on board I fully accountable and committed.

I committed knowing that I would not the full detail in one shot but allowing people to join my programs and try for themselves. That would open the door to the real book with recounts of others results and successes. For my commitment with limited to deadlines set my editor to publish on time. I met and beat my deadlines consistently. Finally, I pushed past all my obstacles and published a week ahead of schedule. Alone, I would probably be still drafting and proofing to infinitum. Get an external force to move you. That is the push you need to make your plan happen. Some use a group, community or simply an accountability partner in the form of the renewal fitness specialist. Most of all you want to get to a point of starting your journey to a better you…just execute!

Executing a plan does not mean that it must be grand only that it must be. Try and do it. It will not be your masterpiece. It does not have to be. Maybe it will just be the proof you need to prove that you can. You set goals and deadlines. Realistic ones. Find a mentor who will embrace you and give you small consumable changes to immediately implement. Communicate openly and speak up when you want to pick up the pace. Before you know it, you will meet and beat your goals!

Just a little bit every day

To reach your destination, you simply must put one foot in front of the other one. Over the past few weeks we have been working on changing our perspective and mindset. Have you been taking these steps? *Setting a Foundation, Mindset, Commit, Plan and Execute*

This is the point where you connect the dots and walk on that journey. Sometimes it feels like you are spinning your wheels. Sometimes your support system will fail or a loved one will fall ill. Teach yourself to overcome and achieve your goals. Be intentional. Step into you purpose a little bit every day. At this point, you are accustomed to making a list of goals and moving towards them.

Start from the inside out. Start your day with affirmations. Look yourself in the mirror and say out loud, "I will achieve three big goals today." The act of looking at yourself and making a verbal intention makes you accountable to yourself. Say your other affirmations out loud. Show yourself that you believe in you. Prevail no matter the obstacles. Saying is where you begin. Continue by stepping into the reality of your belief.

Make your intention known. Email your accountability partner or call them if you are struggling with a goal. Being accountable to yourself is only half the battle but to put your goals on display will push you further. Align yourself with someone who will propel you. Having a partner, coach or community will give you a forum to make your goals known. The positivity and synergy will propel you.

Make your action items big. That means to make the list short and achievable not more than three big items per day and work hard to be accountable to yourself to get it done each day. If your obstacle is knowledge, make your intention to learn something new every day.

> **"Learn what to do and how to do it".**
>
> **T. Harv Eker**

Workout Around My Day is all about doing just a little bit every day. It is about putting one foot in front of the other and learning what and how to do it. It is about believing in yourself and your ability to overcome obstacles of all kinds. In doing so you are setting a foundation and mindset to commit, plan and execute just a little bit every day.

Let's Talk Numbers: Calories, BMI and the Scale

Before I tell you what the experts say, just for a moment think on a few things. Do you know how many calories your body burns in a day? I do not know. Briefly in one of my one of my nutrition classes, we did case studies measuring our calories output and intake. However, most of us could not be accurate for one reason or another. In the end, we were taught that it was a best estimation. An estimation? It gets better the calorie counts on our food labels are also an approximation and placed there to meet FDA requirements. In most cases, the actual count is 20% higher. Not only that all calories are not created equally because different foods are metabolized different in the body.

The overall conclusion amongst experts, doctors in the field of nutrition and heads of nutritional organizations, is that weight gain is due to insulin imbalance, a hormone that balances sugar. The solution is to eat whole nutritious foods which are slow-digesting like fruits, vegetables, chicken, legumes and fats like olive oil not counting calories.

Where it all gets, confusing is when you ask your regular R.D. or registered dietician and some tell you yes and some tell you no. I would call RD's non-experts. We will look at all opinions here.

What do the experts think?

Dr. Robert Lustig, director of the Weight Assessment for Teen and Child Health (WATCH) Program at the University of California, San Francisco and also author of *Fat Chance: Beating the Odds Against Sugar, Processed Food, Obesity, and Disease* says, "Different foods are metabolized differently, absorbed differently, converted into fat or energy differently and raise or lower your risk for disease differently," he says. Focusing on calories ignores all of this complexity".

What is he saying here? The composition of the food that eat determines how your body uses it. A bowl of oatmeal with no toppings or added sugar is 130 calories and a 12 oz. can of a coke has 140 calories. Clearly the oatmeal provides dietary fiber, phosphorus, magnesium, some protein and slowing carbohydrates. Eating a bowl of oatmeal in a rush for breakfast far exceeds the nutritional benefits of a can of coke. However, sometimes people will select liquid calories to give them a boost. The can of coke has 39 g of sugars and 45 mg of sodium. In the body, this type of sugar is immediately stored as fat especially if it replaces breakfast. After sleeping all night, your body needs at minimum a bowl of oatmeal with one tablespoon of coconut oil, in season fruit for slow releasing sugar to elevate the blood sugar to stable and make all system go. Skipping breakfast or selecting liquid alternatives such as soda or rich coffee drinks dehydrates the body, stores fat, gives a false boost, and prolongs the starvation period starting from your last meal, i.e. dinner to your next meal. Extended period of starvation confuses it and elevates a stress response putting it into survival mode. That means next time you eat it will seek the fat first. Why fat? Fat is the building blocks of the nervous systems and while you are in survival mode all systems go haywire especially central control or the brain.

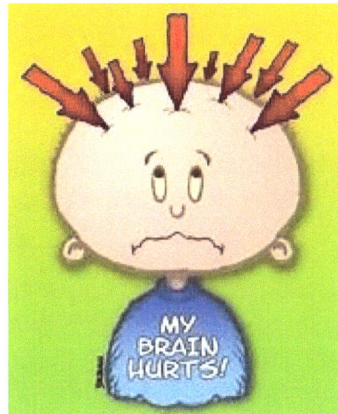

Dr. David Ludwig, a professor of nutrition at the Harvard School of Public Health.

 "People think overeating makes you fat, when really it's the process of getting fat that makes you overeat," says.

Huh? What did he just say? So, in the above example, this person skipped breakfast for a can of coke. Now she is eating half of a sandwich and soup for lunch and a lemonade. It does not seem like much and you are right. It is not much. So now she will begin grazing all day. A bag of chips there, an apple there, a café mocha, a mini candy bar…you get the idea. Maybe a few cups of water in between. Then finally a late dinner of pasta and meat sauce with cheese. The portion will be disproportionate because she has starved herself all day and now the body needs more. Several weeks, months and years of this eating pattern will make you remain in a permanent starvation cycle and overeat.

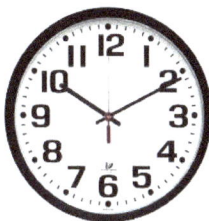

hours go by without a bite and then eat everything in sight

Dr. Marion Nestle, a professor of food and nutrition at New York University and author of *Why Calories Count*

From a basic accounting standpoint, "calorie counting simply can't be done accurately."

This quote resonates with me the most because his argument is the same as Dr. Lustig. It also explains why most of my nutrition class colleagues and I could not seem to get it right. Add in the facts stated on the FDA web site that most calories listed on packaging is an approximation and you have a full argument against calorie counting period. Combined with the state expert's statement:

Dr. Walter Willett, who chairs the Department of Nutrition at Harvard

> **"The quality of our calories, meaning the types of food we eat, has an important effect on whether we gain or lose body fat...Some foods leave us more satisfied than others, and the insulin response to foods can influence how we metabolize or store these calories."**

Now if read any fashion or lifestyle magazine, here comes the confusion. These publications interview R.D.s or Registered Dieticians. These are the same people who work with our family doctors or at healthcare facilities in food service. However, they do not nor are they required to a graduate degree in nutrition. They also are not familiar with "*the science of nutrients and how they are digested, absorbed, transported, metabolized, stored, and eliminated by the body. Besides studying how food works in the body, nutritionists are interested in how the environment affects the quality and safety of foods, and what influence these factors have on health and disease*", according to the University of Maryland Medical Center.

I read an article that interviewed two registered dieticians and one tells us that we should count calories and the other says that we should not. The argument for counting calories is that it provides structure and goals towards building a meal plan. The argument against counting calories is one says that it is a losing battle because it is impossible to capture every calorie that goes into your mouth." These contradictions in mass media confuse and perpetuate misinformation resulting in diabetes, heart failure, cancer and obesity. That is why, I encourage women especially mothers to charge of their health as pillars of the family. Our children learn from our choices, habits and the subliminal messages surrounding food.

BMI – What Does It Mean?

First, per most experts, "body mass index is an imperfect measure of mortality" and factors such as blood pressure, cholesterol and blood sugar should be considering to measure overall health, said Dr. Samuel Klein, Director of the Center for Human Nutrition at Washington University School of Medicine, St. Louis. (nytimes.com, January 1, 2013, "Study Suggest Lower Mortality Risks for People Deemed to be Overweight"). In a 1912 study, the example of a perfect woman was 5'7" and 171 pounds. That means that she had a BMI of about 27 or clinically overweight. The shake out of these studies suggest that fat in youth during your adolescence and in your senior years can be protective if well placed. Of course, most concur that belly fat is detrimental to health because it causes diabetes, heart failure, cancer and the list goes on. Some even believe that the scales of BMI should be revised to exclude the lower, underweight category of people. In the case of the perfect woman, she lived to be 91 years old.

I say that it is all relative and the numbers to pay attention to are cholesterol, blood sugar and blood pressure. Between annual check-ups, pay attention to use of salt, sugar and serving portion per meal. Most of all know your limits and your body. You know when you are doing your body good and when you are abusing it. Measuring yourself per societal standards of beauty will always

Definition

Body Mass Index (BMI) is a person's weight in kilograms divided by the square of height in meters. A high BMI can be an indicator of high body fatness.

In general, BMI is an inexpensive and easy-to-perform method of screening for weight category, for example underweight, normal or healthy weight, overweight, and obesity.

How is BMI used?

A high BMI can be an indicator of high body fatness. BMI can be used as a screening tool but is not diagnostic of the body fatness or health of an individual.

To determine if a high BMI is a health risk, a healthcare provider would need to perform further assessments. These assessments might include skinfold thickness measurements, evaluations of diet, physical activity, family history, and other appropriate health screenings[10].

Cdc.org

diminish your opinion of self. Instead, don't worry about the numbers, love the body you are in with daily self-love rituals. Smiling at yourself will reduce stress, relax your muscle and lower your blood pressure. It brings clarity and gives you hope and prevents wrinkles. Fact: It takes less muscles to smile than to frown.

The Truth About the Scale

You may not even know your body mass index or never cared but you probably find yourself hovering over your scale regularly.

As we age, the numbers on the scale become less true. Our body composition shifts so much between, pregnancies, gravity, muscle tone and inflammation the scale often does not give us the full picture.

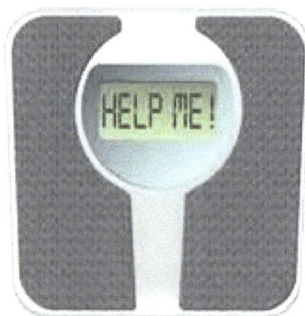

" Oh no! I gained another pound!"

Knowing how much you weigh is only part of the story. In fact, I tell my clients to only weigh once a month just to get an idea of progress. Most often if you want to know changes are happening, grab your measuring tape. Your proportions are what make your clothes fit or too snug not your weight. If you have started weight training, you may gain weight before losing it. Muscle weighs more and it takes time to burn off the fat between the muscle. Once you are in a habit of weight training however, your body will become a fat burning machine even if you miss a few days. Consider your eating habits and seasoning choices. How much salt are you eating? As little as ½ teaspoon of salt can retain up to 16 ounces of water. That is one pound. Sugar causes inflammation in the joints. How has the weather been lately? Rainy and overcast weather can cause up to six pounds of water retention or even just a low -pressure stream can make you retain fluid.

Bear in mind 34,000 people per year die from being underweight and being slightly overweight is not all that bad as we have already seen. During the winter, it is also normal to gain up to ten pounds as protection. These are unavoidable human genetic conditions so that we can survive. Girls entering puberty will also gain 10 – 20 pounds which they will shed once in their twenties. I distinctly remember this and am now seeing that with my own daughters. Your daughters and sons are watching you and are learning about loving their bodies through you.

How Our Choices Effect Our Children?

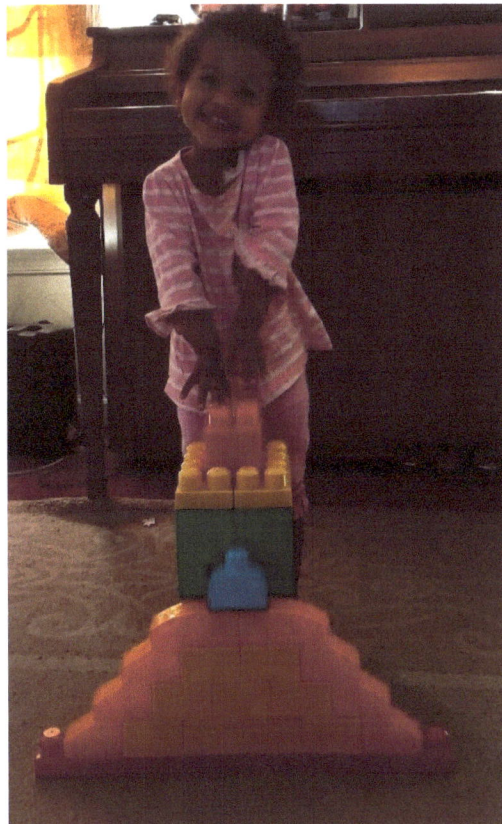

We have examined our choices but not how it effects our innocent observers...yes our children. They are learning mindset and habits surrounding food by watching us. Picky eaters are making a choice. If you skip breakfast or lunch or graze, they are observing and choosing to be just like you. Early on when they are very young, they may not say it but you will eventually hear, "Well you never eat breakfast!" or "Why can't we eat like everyone else? I want Mc Donald's!" Ultimately, we want our children to fall somewhere in the middle of these two statements. What is the balance in raising happy healthy children?

On the next page, I will expound on ten points. I can simply sum it up to say enjoy her joy and successes. Above is a picture taken by my older son of my youngest daughter. They had worked together on building this castle. She stacked what she could and directed him where she could not. Sometimes it is easier for an older sibling to encourage and be the cheerleader. I was pleased to see the outcome of their project and how my son selflessly gave all the credit to his little sister. I was a little jealous also because I wished it had been my project with her. In a way, it was because if I had not raised him the way he is; then, he would not have been there to empower her for me.

Raising Happy Healthy Children

1. Love and appreciate them for who they are

Each child is a small individual who is shaping an opinion and set of behaviors towards the world as they experience. We as parents can guide, facilitate, redirect, empower but not control the outcome. Sometimes your child can be your best teacher. Be humbled as they grow and develop.

2. Breastfeeding sets gut flora and children are less likely to be obese. The milk is made uniquely for each child.

So many studies have been done in favor of extended, over six months, breast feeding. Personally, I have nursed all six of mine and the healthier more confident ones were nursed the longest.

3. Mindset that develops in a breastfed child is one of abundance. No fear of lack.

One thing about my children that is lovable and exasperating at the same time is there abundance mindset. There is no limit of delicious, nutritious food in the house so I will share with all the neighbors and pack an extra lunch for my friends and you can just go buy more. (Ha-ha, gotta love that within limitation!)

4. **Get them involved in the food selection process whether, by grocery shopping or gardening or cooking meals**

Once my children are about three, they want to active "helpers" at the grocery store so oblige them by letting them collect 8 limes or a bunch of cilantro. In this way, they are learning to count and vegetable identification. They are also excited about what they want to make when we get home. You will have a built-in food preparation crew at meal time. A child that makes his own food will eat it.

5. **If you are integrated in the food decision making you are also fulfilled in your connection to food decision making you are also**

6. **Only buy whole foods. Fresh vegetables, fruits, meats, dry beans, spices, herbs, individual baking ingredients**

7. **Learning by seeing foods in their original form changes the association to food. I teach my children the purpose of each ingredient when we cook and how it provides nutrients to the body.**

8. **Snack time should not be on demand but part of a routine after a physical activity. Like we went for a walk, hike, played at the playground, etc. time for a high protein fatty but hydrating snack like cashews and berries.**

9. **Food association should have purpose like a mathematical equation.**

10. **Be a role model by loving you because that is how they will learn to love themselves.**

Healthy Hosting, Holiday, and Social Eating

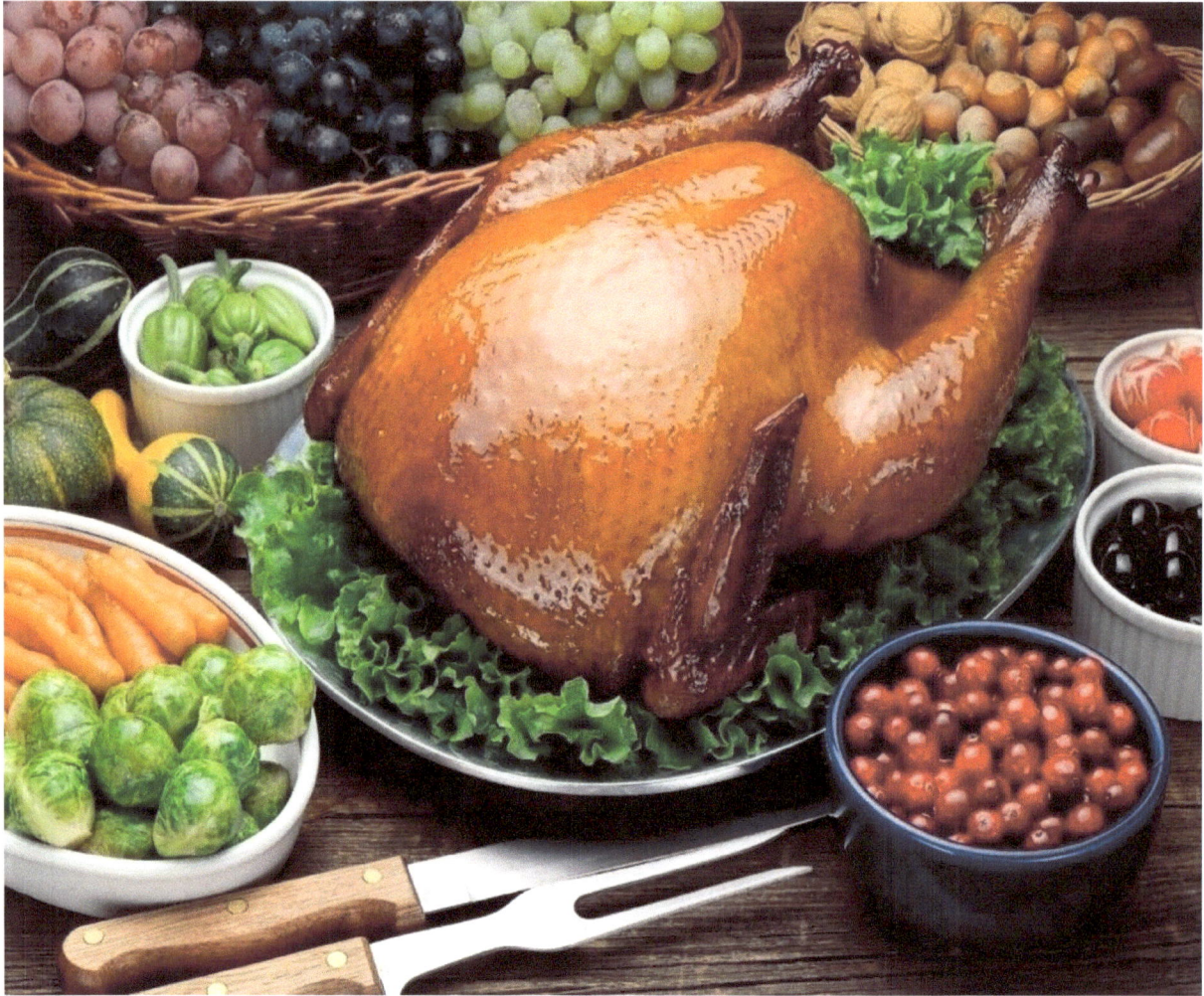

Turkey dinner

Everything that you can normally stay away from is waiting for you at that holiday gathering. You want to be polite or just splurge because you are socializing. Cake and bread and cookies never tasted so good. Why not just have one soft drink? Social eating is normal in the summer and during holidays. Enjoy have a good time but stay on track. How can you have the best of both worlds? I will show you how to eat your cake and have it too.

Above the host has great options-fresh fruits, nuts, steamed vegetables, baked turkey with fresh greens and no stuffing or gravy in sight. Most often the host or hostess does not make it so easy to select choices.

Making good choices in life is easy with no temptations. How do you stay away from that great homemade cake by your Aunt Ophelia? You don't have to. Have a slice but just one. It is all about the timing, portion and order.

Timing. Start by eating well before leaving home and drinking water throughout the day. By eating a well-balanced meal with slowing sugars and being hydrated before leaving home you solve three issues:

1. You will not be hungry and will be able to make wise decisions
2. When you eat, the nutrients will be absorbed first instead of the fats or other empty calories
3. Usually we think that we are hungry when in fact we are thirsty.

What that looks like is a protein and fat based with fiber. Now in English.

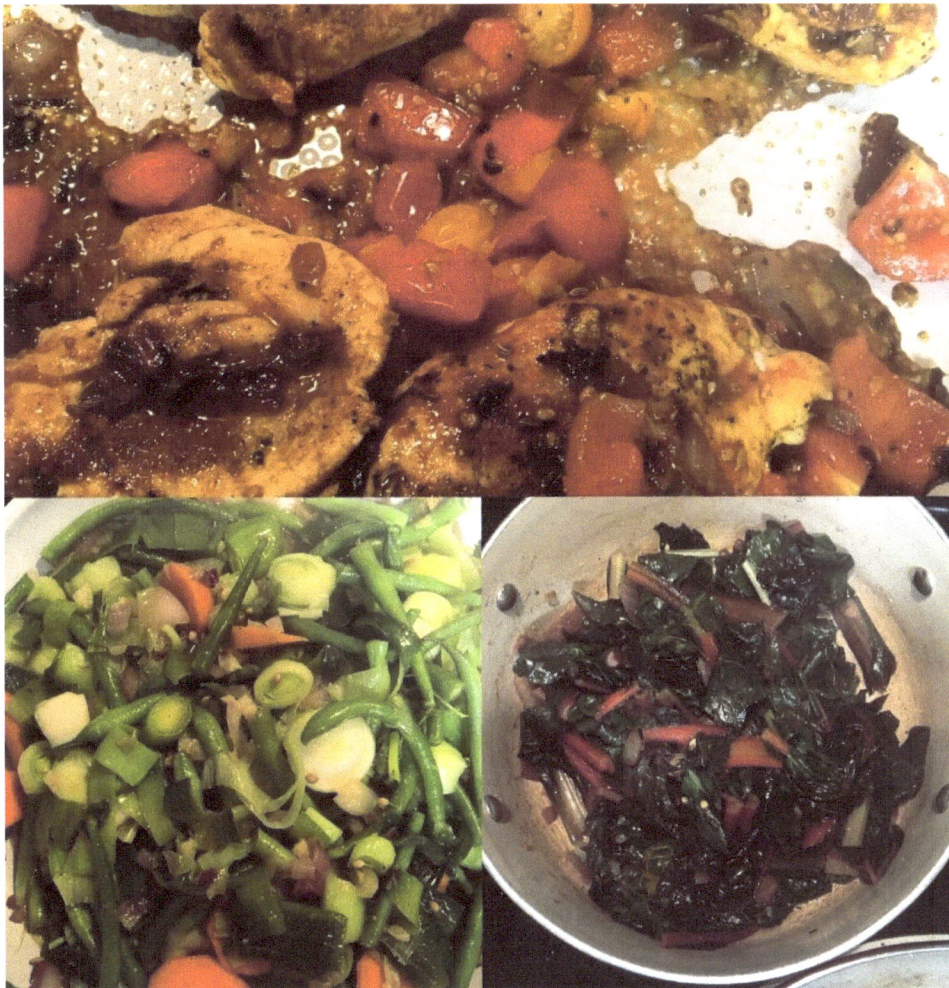

At the top, sautéed curry chicken. Left bottom, steamed leeks, carrots and string beans. Right bottom, rainbow swiss chard mixed with dandelion.

This is the perfect pre-holiday gathering meal. You have a balance of animal and plant based protein (dandelion), spices and seasoning to prep the body for digesting (turmeric, cumin, black pepper, garlic, red and green onions, and ginger. Fiber and carbs are in the carrots and beans. (All recipes in the bonus recipe section under dinner) Alternatively, if you do not have access to this, at minimum have the leeks, beans and carrots sautéed in coconut oil with green onion, garlic, ginger, black pepper and a dash of Himalayan salt over a palm full of quinoa rice mix.

That may solve the eating issue but what about drinks, you may be thinking. Take

> **Although men are more likely to drink alcohol and drink in larger amounts, gender differences in body structure and chemistry cause women to absorb more alcohol, and take longer to break it down and remove it from their bodies (i.e., to metabolize it). In other words, upon drinking equal amounts, women have higher alcohol levels in their blood than men, and the immediate effects of alcohol occur more quickly and last longer in women than men. These differences also make it more likely that drinking will cause long-term health problems in women than men.**
>
> Cdc.org

half a cup of your favorite sweet beverage and cut it with the bottle of water you brought or available. And your favorite cocktail being offered by your best friend? I will explain it this way. One glass of white wine will stay increase your weight by five pounds and stay on you for a week. See the box with information on the CDC web site.

Remember that alcohol is made from sugar. Hard liquor is a product from molasses, sometimes wheat barley and wine from grapes. Be mindful when drinking and indulging in sugary treats, salty or even fatty foods.

Portion. At the beginning of the book we discussed portion in detail and even did a portion control challenge. Apply those rules, perhaps review them before going out. Maybe you would have even mastered them before going out. The point is on social occasions partake in moderation. Here is how to ensure that it does not make a downward spiral on your health.

1. First always drink plenty of water before going to a party or event. Most often a limited supply of water will be available. Hydration is cumulative so make sure the days leading up the occasion and the day of you are drinking more than enough water
2. Hydration is half the battle. If you feel full, you will eat and drink less.
3. Keep moving and when you are standing don't eat or drink. When you are thirsty or hungry sit down.

Order.
1. When first arrive eat the protein and fat options, like nuts, finger sized portions of meat appetizers or pack a protein bar like Pro bar.
2. Then indulge in the carbohydrate options like pasta dishes, potatoes and rice.
3. Finally, now that your body is well nourished you may drink sweet drinks and alcohol if you choose or have any other sweets like cakes, pies and cookies. Wash it all down with water and try to break up your eating with at least half cup of water.

Getting back on track. Don't wait for tomorrow. Clean your system when you get home. Drink a warm cup of water or chamomile tea when you return home. If you are hungry or have space, have a 6-ounce cup of plain organic yogurt with chia seeds. Yogurt should only have two ingredients: whole organic milk and live cultures. There should be at least four live cultures: B. Lactis, L. Acidophillus, L. Delbrueckii, bulgaricus, and S. Thermophillus. Make sure to read your labels. The yogurt will cleanse your gut flora and will act as natural probiotics in your system. The chia seeds will purge any excess. Dr. Oz says, "The tryptophan in chia seeds, like in turkey, raises melatonin and serotonin levels, which promotes stable sleep. With more than twice the tryptophan of turkey, you'll need just 2 ounces of chia seeds to help you snooze." Two ounces is one tablespoon.

Exercise as soon as you get out of bed. Start your day with a cleansing workout. Do a low impact Pilates workout or a short weight bearing HIIT (high intensity interval training) workout? This will oxygenate your whole system and force toxins out. It will also restart your metabolism. The message sent to your muscle, lungs and brain is reject all toxins and activate metabolism.

Eat well immediately following. Get right back to having a well-balanced diverse breakfast. After eating sugary and heavy foods, I usually am very hungry the next morning. Your body is starved of actual nutrition. Give it fresh in season organic fruits and vegetables, wholesome sources of protein like boiled eggs, fava beans, quinoa or oatmeal.

Don't deny yourself at social events.

- Nourish and Hydrate before you go and while you are there
- While there, be mindful of timing, portion and order
- Cleanse when you get home
- Exercise the next morning
- Feed your body the proper nutrition following workout

MINDFUL INDULGENCE

· *NOURISH AND HYDRATE BEFORE YOU GO*

· *WHILE THERE, BE MINDFUL OF TIMING, PORTION AND ORDER*

· *CLEANSE WHEN YOU GET HOME*

· *EXERCISE THE NEXT MORNING*

· *FEED YOUR BODY THE PROPER NUTRITION FOLLOWING WORKOUT*

Now How to be a Healthy Hostess

1 – Offer healthy food choices – Use the highest quality meat such as grass fed beef and free range chicken. Organic condiments or better alternatives. Instead of ketchup simply organic tomatoes or sundried tomatoes; instead of mayonnaise cucumbers in grass fed yogurt with salt and pepper. Think outside of the box. Instead of mustard or pickles use organic cucumbers or olive oil oven roasted sweet peppers.

2- Have pure fresh water available – Have fresh spring water delivered and use reusable cups and a sharpie. (The sharpie is to write the names of your guest). Most parties are short on fresh water. Do yourself and your guest a favor save some money and have water delivered. It is less expensive than carbonated choices. Not just where cups are concerned as much as possible think about the environment. I know it is a lot to have a party but use the higher quality reusable plastic cups, plates and ware if possible.

3- Have healthy sweet drink alternatives (homemade soda) – Put your soda maker to work and make a variety of less sweet less carbonated preservative free soda. Also, make fresh squeezed juice options using less sugar and combining a pinch of sea salt for more hydration with your fresh spring water.

4- Limited alcoholic beverages – Make it the theme of the party when you announce. This is a one drink party or alternative alcohol party. You will save money and limit liquid calories for everyone.

5- Healthier desert options – A regular cut into 27 squares topped with one scoop of grass fed yogurt (it is creamier and thicker), 2-3 raspberries, sprinkled hemp seeds and walnuts. Melons and tropical fruits are another great option. Below is a picture where, I topped the yogurt with goji berries.

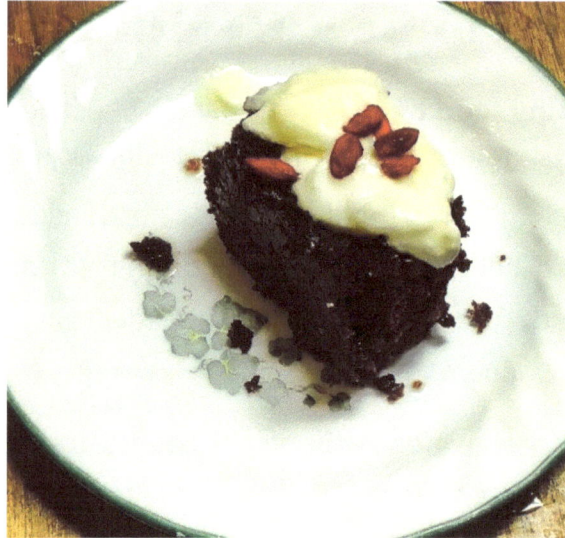

6- Fruit platters with high vitamins C and hydrating – Beyond oranges, grapefruits and limes we have a world of hydrating fruits high in vitamin C. Papaya, pineapple, kiwi, mango and cantaloupe make a delightful and nutritious fruit platter.

7- Vegetable platters and salads – Here is a complimenting list of vegetables that are both hydrating and high in vitamin C. The importance of vitamin C in foods is to boost the immune system and work as a stimulant replacing caffeine drinks like soda, coffees or teas. Some great choices are: bell peppers, broccoli and cauliflower.

8- Marinade meats days in advance or the night before – Seasoning meats and <u>fish</u> overnight make them more flavorful and with the right herbs such as cilantro, garlic and cumin can prevent salmonella poisoning.

9 – Bake the burgers before grilling- Seems crazy, right? The whole point of cooking outside is to keep the heat out of the kitchen. However, you want to avoid serving raw red meat. Ten minutes in the oven on 375 F will also seal in the flavor, which is the reason for the pre-bake.

10 – Cook meats separately – Another way to avoid food poisoning is to cover the grill with new foil every time you change the type of meat being cooked. Just cook each meat separately.

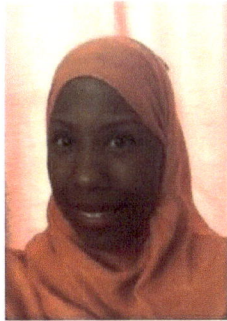

5 Tips to Stay Fit During Winter

1. SELECT SOUP OR BONE BROTH OVER SWEETS

2- STAY HYDRATED

3- DRINK GREEN TEA

4- EAT A BALANCE OF PROTEIN

5- STOP FEEDING INTO YOUR TRIGGERS (SAD)

WWW.WORKOUTAROUNDMYDAY.COM

Thank you for reading you now have all the tools you need to maintain your health.

Practice, apply, try, rinse and repeat!

Bonus Section

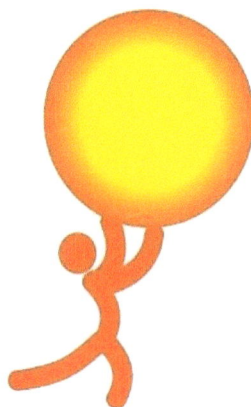

A Few Recipes
toGetStarted
Cooking with

WORKOUT

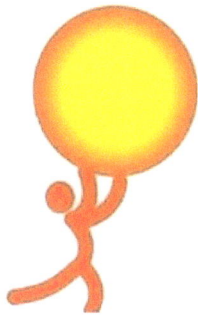

AROUND
MY DAY

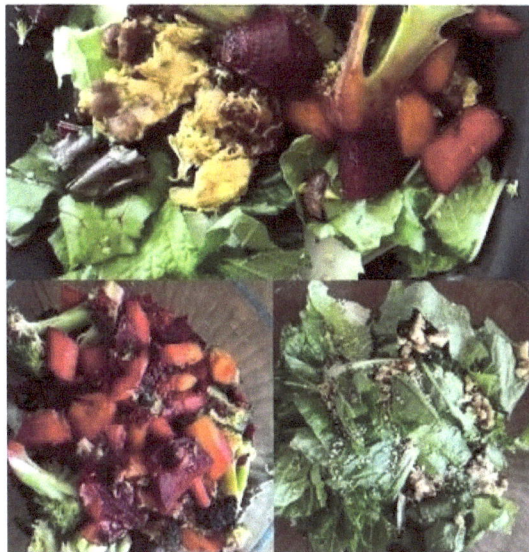

The blend of cultural flavors and beliefs shows how much all humanity shares!

Thanksgiving dinner is always a treat. When I prepare for my extended family that are Bengali, Egyptian and Arab. Being of Cherokee, Scottish and African Caribbean mix, I pull from the wealth cultural flavors available in my chef's mind. Not to mention my crunchy, earth conscientious, health minded side. That means Tandoori Turkey, corn pudding made with organic vanilla yogurt, seasonal blend of bitter greens flavored with ginger and Himalayan salt, wild rice made with organic brown rice mixed with quinoa and the hottest crush red peppers in the world tamed with organic coconut milk, stuffing, dripping gravy, sweet potato casserole, pasta casserole and of course cranberry sauce. Every year I try a new recipe with the cranberry sauce always fresh cranberries but sometimes with pomegranate to boost the immune system.

In these few pages, I am sharing the blends of deliciousness that I have created to maintain our health whilst tantalizing our palate. From breakfast to desert and the meals in between even the snacks are a creative endeavor. Use these ideas to get back on track or to start you cooking journey. There are old favorites with a twist and new flavors with an old-fashioned aroma. You will be transported to your grandma's kitchen and propelled to the latest mid-town hot spot.

Some staples to keep on hand:

Oatmeal

Eggs

Fresh in season fruits and vegetables

Nuts

Sunflower seeds

Chia seeds

Plain grass fed yogurt

Golden berries, goji berries, figs and dates

Dry beans or organic canned BPA free beans

Local grass fed meat and poultry, Spices, garlic, ginger, cilantro

THE RECIPES

- BREAKFAST
- LUNCH
- SNACKS
- DINNER
- DESERT

BREAKFAST

- OATMEAL
- EGG DISHES
- SMOOTHIES

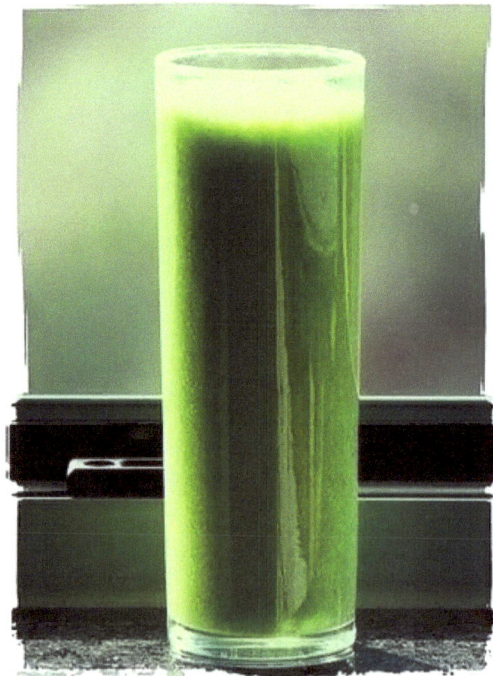

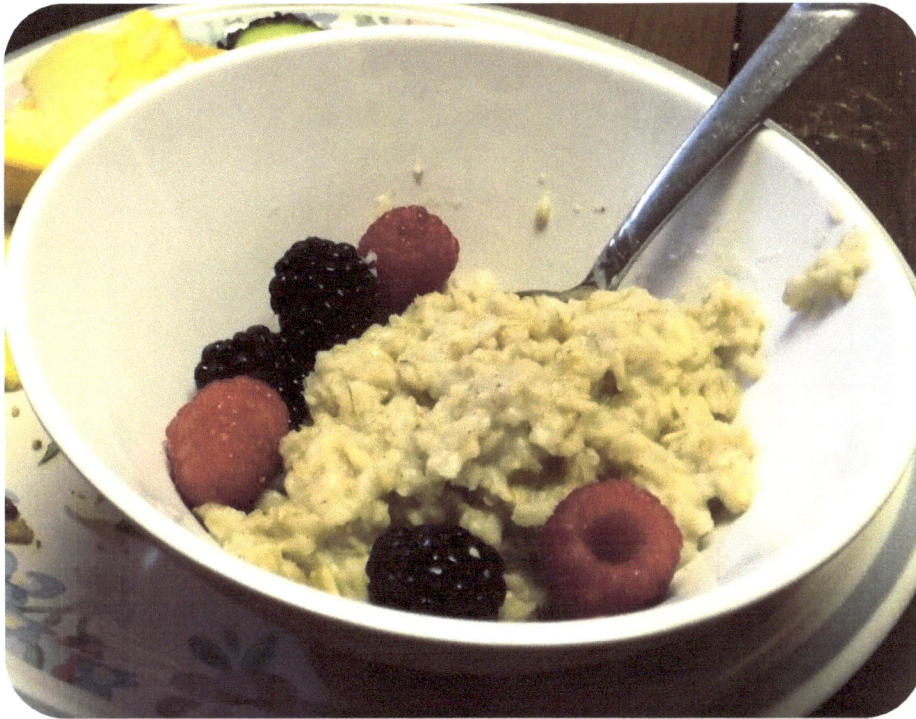

- Oatmeal or Rolled oats

- Berries or other in season fruits

- ½ tbsp. coconut oil

- Chia seeds

- Mashed nuts (pistachios, walnuts or almonds)

Cooking instructions:

Microwave portion by the bowl or on stove top following package instructions

Add in season fruits for sweetener

½ tbsp. of coconut or walnut oil

Sprinkle chia seeds or crushed nuts (walnuts, pistachios or almonds)

Fresh Garden Egg Wrap

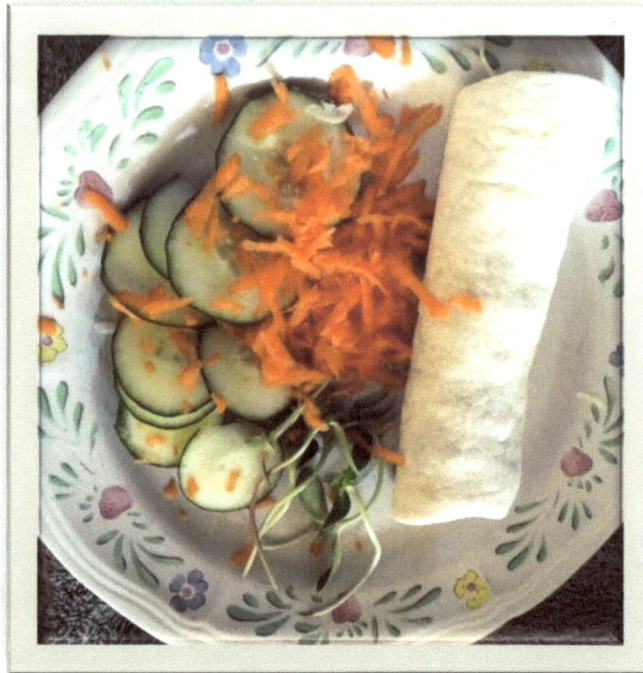

-
- Serves 5
- 5 eggs
- 1 TBSP sharp cheddar or goat cheese
- Grated carrots
- Fresh cucumbers
- Fresh salad greens
- One tortilla or another wrap
- Coconut oil
- (optional) pinch of Pink Himalayan salt

Cooking instructions:

Fava Beans and boiled eggs

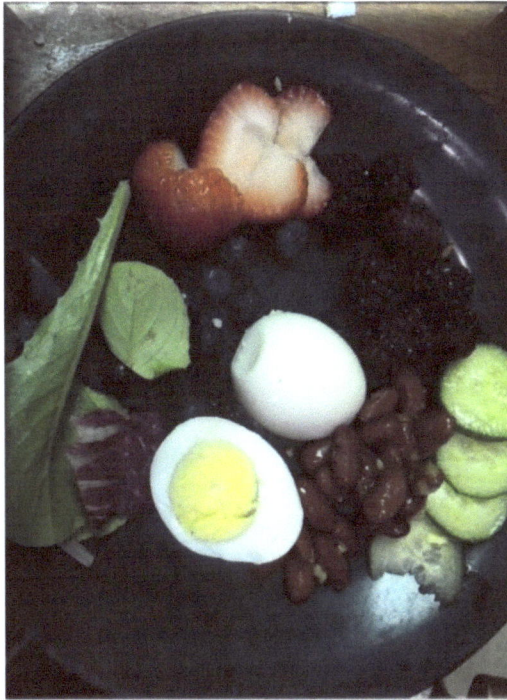

- Serves one

- Two boiled eggs

- One spoon of fava beans

- Fresh salad greens

- Cucumbers

- Blue berries

- Blackberries

- Strawberries

- Note: May substitute other in season fruits

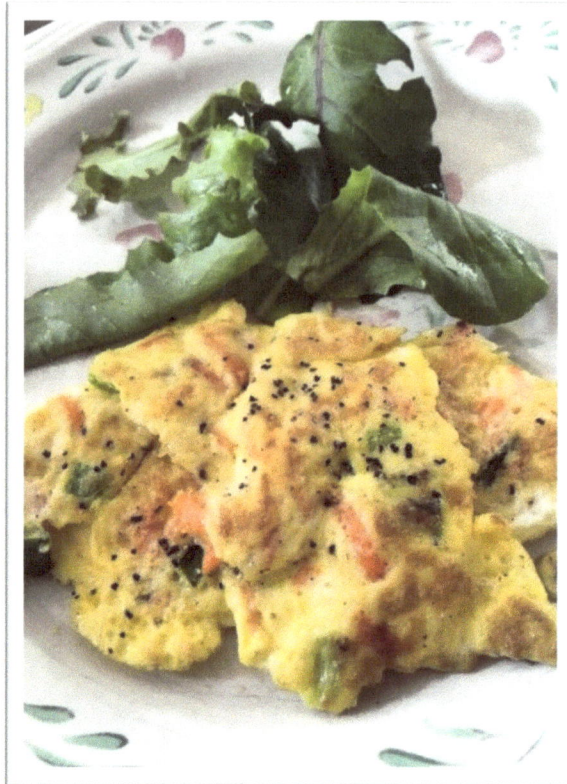

Omelet with cheese and vegetables

This variation is for those sensitive to raw carrots.

5 eggs

black pepper

dash of Himalayan salt

¼ - ½ shredded organic carrots

1/3 cup shredded white sharp cheddar cheese

Scramble ingredients

Pour into a pan with coconut oil and cook them flip and serve with fresh salad greens or cilantro.

Energizing Smoothie

This is a quick and easy high protein drink to start your day!

Ingredients:

¾ cup	Coconut water or coconut milk
1 TBSP	Wheat germ
2 tsp	Hemp seeds
1 ½ tsp	Brewers' yeast
2 TBSP	Maple Syrup
1	Ground flax seeds
1	Orange peeled, seeded and sectioned with pulp
1	Banana, peeled and sliced
1/8 tsp	Nutmeg
2	Ice cubes

1. Add all ingredients into the blender.
2. Blend at the top speed for one minute until completely mixed and frothy.
3. Makes two 8 oz. servings. One for morning and one for mid-afternoon.

Nourishing Smoothie

This is a quick and easy high protein drink to start the day.

Ingredients:

¾ cup	Coconut water or coconut milk
2 cups	Bok Choy (just the greens)
1	Anjou Pear
1/3 cup	Rolled oats
1 TBSP	Coconut oil
½	Ground cinnamon
1	Avocado

1. Blend liquid and greens until smooth.
2. Add the remaining ingredients; blend until smooth.
3. Use frozen fruit to make cold.
4. Makes two 8 oz. servings. One for morning and one for mid-afternoon.

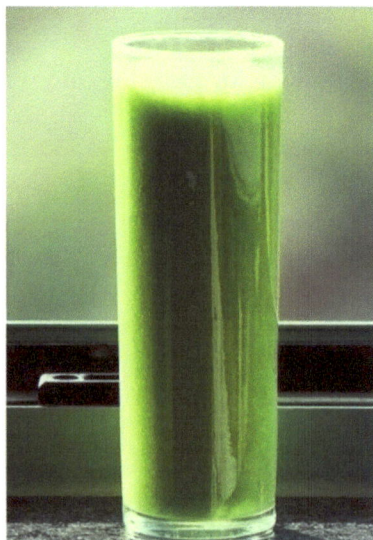

LUNCH

- SALADS
- SANDWICHES
- ENTREES

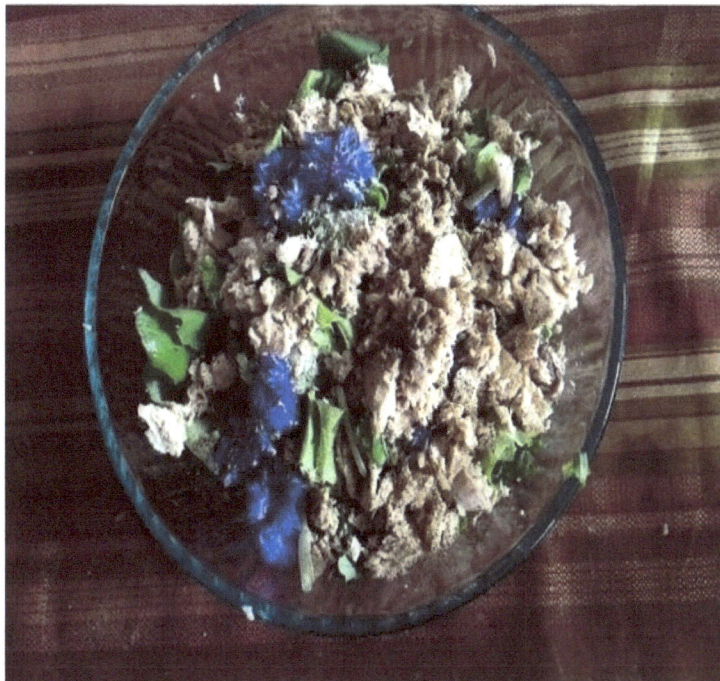

Before we get into lunch and dinner, here is a short cut for seasoning your fish, chicken and meat. Lamb is also another great source of nutrition. In all cases, make sure that you get grass-fed, non-GMO fed, non- chemically treated (hormones, etc.) meat. In fact, while I do not recommend you becoming vegan during pregnancy, limit your meat intake to two to three times per week and only 4-6 ounces per meal. The reason for this is that meat can cause the body to become acidic. This manifest in the form of inflammation, pain, discomfort and lethargy. When eating meat, it is also important to help your body to digest it with certain spices like ginger, garlic, cumin, cinnamon, turmeric and cilantro also known as coriander. Additionally, vegetables like bok choy, beets, carrots and potatoes will help your body to assimilate the fats and proteins in the meat.

You are probably thinking, that is great information but who has time to cook all that? So here I purchase chicken or turkey breast and stew pieces of lamb. You can buy spice mixes that include these herbs just read the labels. Cilantro, ginger and garlic you can buy fresh. Take these ingredients and make a paste in the blender and store. When you buy, the meat wash it and pull out your spice paste and marinade it. Freeze it in a Ziploc bag for later. When you are ready to cook it, just defrost and throw into the pressure cooker advertised on my web site www.workoutaroundmyday.com. Press the settings for meat and an hour you have a meal. It also has settings for rice, pasta and vegetables.

Here is a sample paste recipe:

2 bulbs of garlic, skinned and crushed

1 4- inch piece of skinned and chopped ginger

½ bunch of cilantro

¼ cup of water

1. Place in a blender or large food processer.
2. Blend on high until it makes a watery paste.
3. Store in a mason jar.
4. Use as needed.

KNOW YOUR OILS

HIGH HEAT FRYING
AVOCADO 570F
RICE BRAN OIL 490 F

LOW TO MEDIUM HEAT
SAUTE AND STEAMING
COCONUT OR OLIVE OIL
SESAME OR PEANUT
SWEET ALMOND OIL

RAW
FOR VINGARETTE OR
OTHER USE
WALNUT
OLIVE
AVOCADO
GRAPESEED

Sample spice mix recipe:

Per two pounds of meat your mix should have the following. You can either premix and store for later just multiply the recipe depending on how much meat you will cook that week.

2 TBSP turmeric powder

3 TBSP Cumin powder

½ tsp red pepper

½ tsp black pepper

1 teaspoon cinnamon

1 teaspoon fennel seed

Notice that I did not mention salt. Salt should be added the day that you are cooking directly to the meat before putting the mixture. Only use a dash of pink Himalayan salt. Himalayan salt has medicinal value and gives more nutrition when added during cooking.

Now you have your paste and spice mixes ready. Wash your meat marinade it (using your paste and spice mix) and freeze to cook later that same week or get started today. This is also a task that you can delegate or coordinate with your partner or spouse. We will touch on enlisting the help of others.

Did You Know?

Himalayan Salt is made up primarily of sodium and contains 60 to 65 trace minerals. Sodium helps keep your blood pressure in check as well as aiding in cardiovascular function.

KNOW YOUR OILS

AVOID COOKING WITH:

CANOLA OIL
SOYBEAN OIL
GRAPESEED OIL
SMART BALANCE OIL

CAUTION
(NEVER HIGH HEAT)
SESAME
PEANUT
SWEET ALMOND OIL

Salads are always great quick meals. You can steam carrots, beets, broccoli, and asparagus. Nuts and seeds are great substitutes to meat if you just can't get it done. You will be surprised how filling and nutritious small quantities of impactful foods can be.

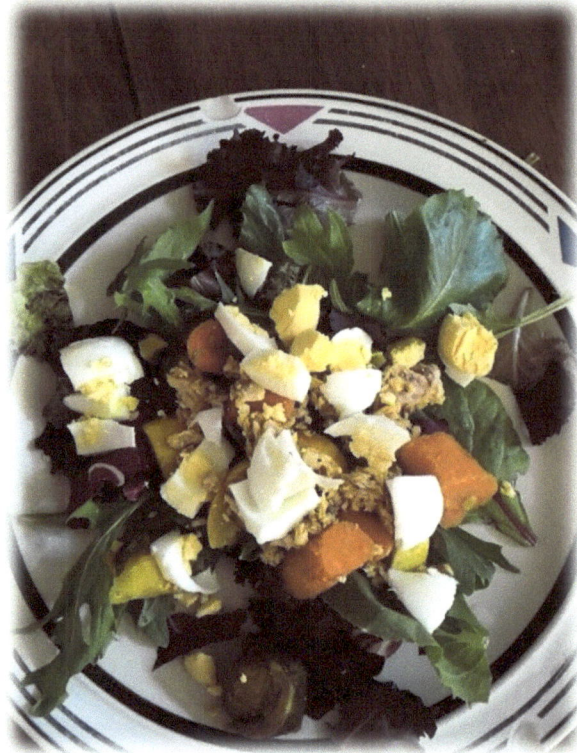

Here we have a mixture of steamed and raw vegetables.

2 boiled eggs

2 large carrots, peeled and sliced

1 cup of wild organic salad mix

1 can of Wild caught Alaskan Salmon

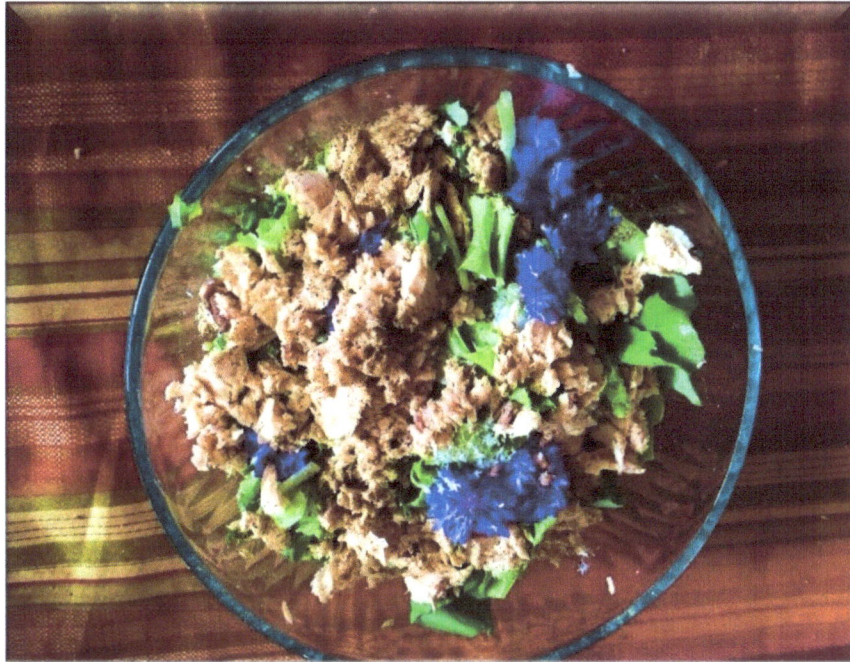

- Wild Alaskan Salmon (canned is fine)

- Sweet White Turnips

- Spring Scallions

- Tender Spring Lettuce Mix

- Bunch of Kale

- Arugula

- Sunflower Sprouts

- Edible Flowers (optional in spring or summer)

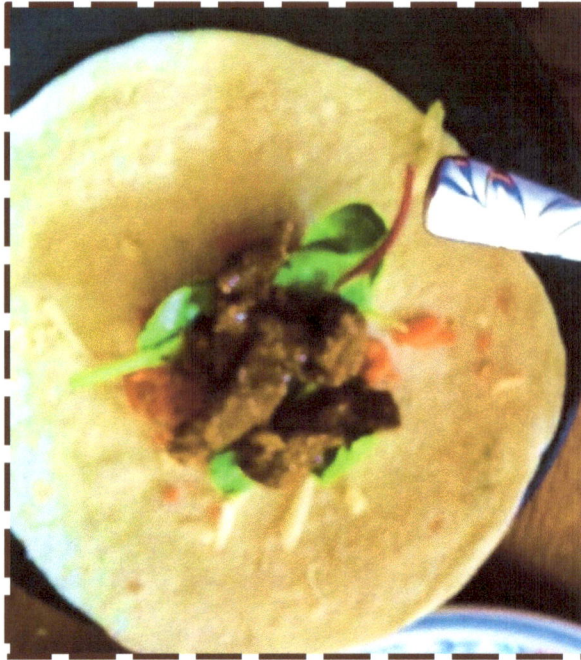

Lunch Meat Wrap

Serves Four

4 tortillas or other flat bread

- Fresh salad greens

- grated carrots

- Grated fresh ginger

- 1 ounce of any leftover meat

- Here used blade steak

- Optional cheese

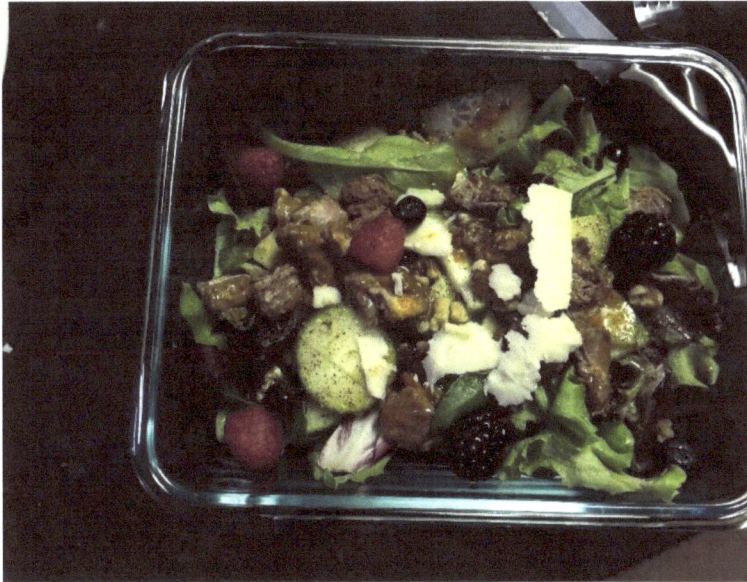

Lamb Curry Salad

- 2 kg Lamb

- 1 TBSP Cumin seeds

- 1 TBSP Turmeric powder

- 2 TBSP Paprika powder

- ½ TBSP Cinnamon powder

- ½ tsp Clove powder

- 2 TBSP Coriander powder

- 1 TBSP Ground black or red pepper

- Ingredients Continued

- 2 TSBP Coconut or avocado oil

- 7-8 minced cloves of garlic

- 1 finely chopped

- green onion/ scallion

- 1finely chopped medium red onion

- dash of pink Himalayan salt

- Up to 1 cup of water

- Ingredients for salad

- Fresh garden cucumber

- Raspberries

- Blue berries

- Blackberries

- Salad greens

- Optional goat cheese or sharp cheddar

- Directions

- 1. Mix all spices together in a small bowl

- 2. Clean stew meat pieces

- 3. Combine spices with meat and set aside to marinate

- 4.In a large sauce pan, turn on low heat and brown cumin seeds.

- 5. When lightly browned, add oil and chopped onions and scallions.

- 6.Mix minced garlic to meat mix

- 7. Once onions are browned add meat and stir

- 8. Cover and continue to cook for an hour stirring and adding up to 1 cup of water as needed.

Can also be placed in a pressure cooker after step 7 only use ½ cup of water.

- Directions Continued

- 9. Place salad greens in a container

- 10. chop or slice cucumber

- 11. clean and place berries

- 12. shred or crumb cheese

13. Optional: Use the sauce from the meat for a topping

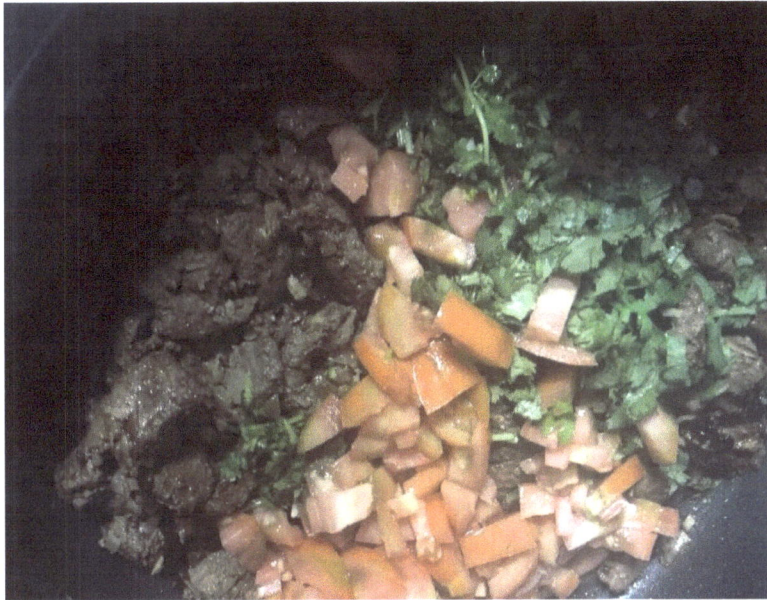

Beef Liver Curry Salad

- Beef liver
  2-3 livers cut in to cubes
  2 medium sized onions chopped (or one large one)
  1 bulb of garlic (7-8 cloves)
  Fresh ginger minced
  2 TBSP curry powder
  1 tsp cinnamon
  1 tsp clove
  1/2 tsp salt
  1 TSBP cumin seeds
  2 large tomatoes chopped
  1/2 bunch of cilantro chopped
  1-2 TBSP of coconut oil
  7-8 small red potatoes chopped

- 1. Warm oil and sauté cumin seeds with onions.
  2. Mix powdered spices and most of garlic and ginger with liver and set aside
  3. Add liver mix once onions are browned

4. Brown on each side on medium heat
5. Add garlic, tomatoes and cilantro
6. Cover on medium low heat stirring regularly
7. Add chopped potatoes and one cup of water
8. Let cook until potatoes are soft.

The process

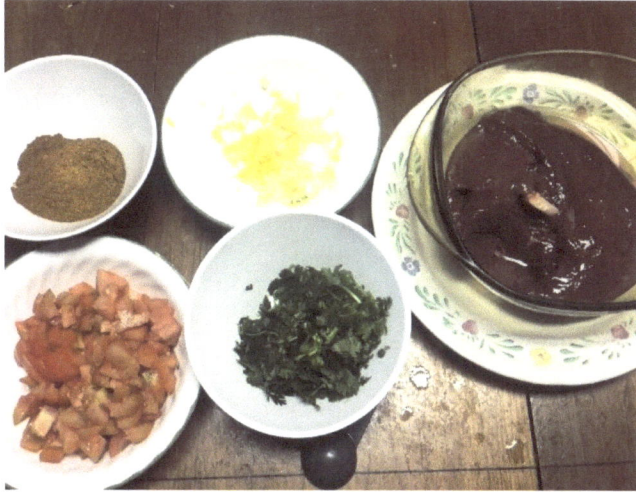

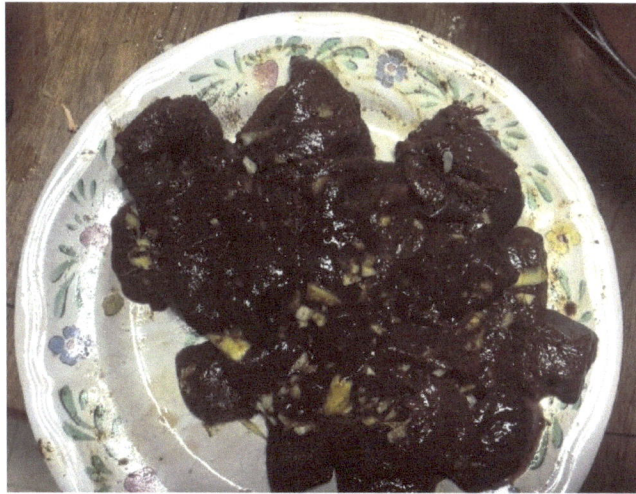

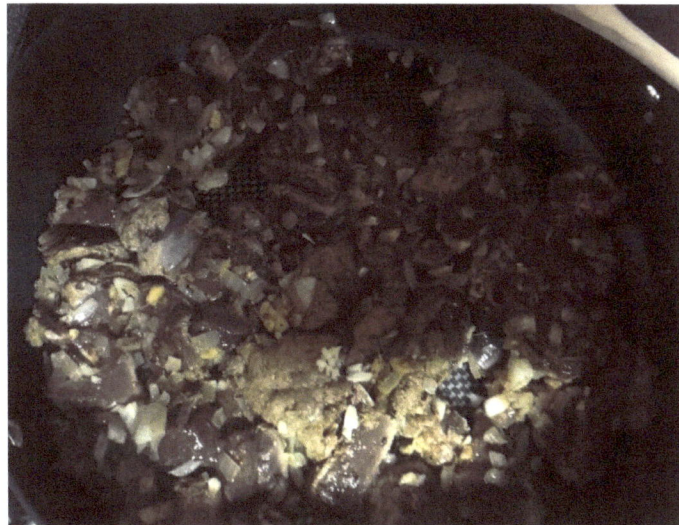

SNACKS

- FRUITS
- DRINKS
- NUTS, SEEDS

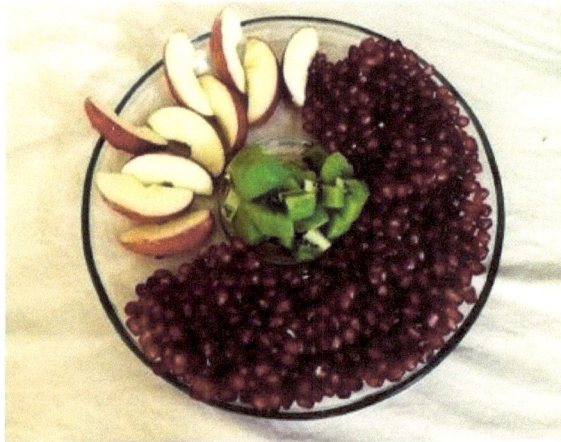

Simplicity in snacks is best. The lighter the better if the choices are nutrient dense. Sometimes it could be the leftovers from another meal, like seeds from the pumpkin to make pumpkin pie or the skins from apple or sweet potatoes. It can also be something simple to combine like:

- Yogurt and berries
- Yogurt with chia seeds
- Grass fed whole yogurt or homemade
- 2 TBSP of chia seeds
- Blueberries strawberries
- Dried fruit and nuts
- Seeds and nuts

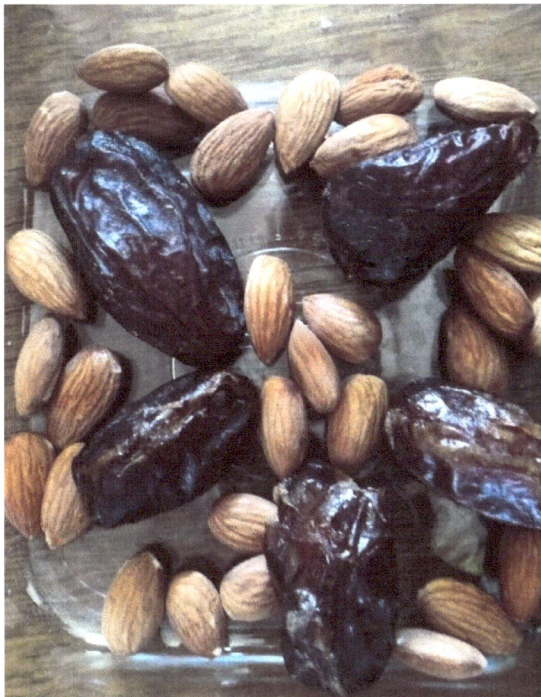

Dates and Almonds

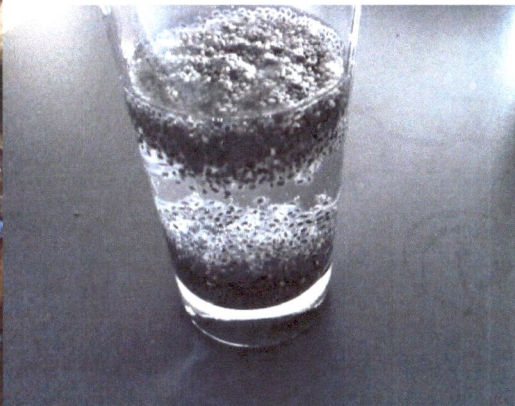

Chia seed water gel

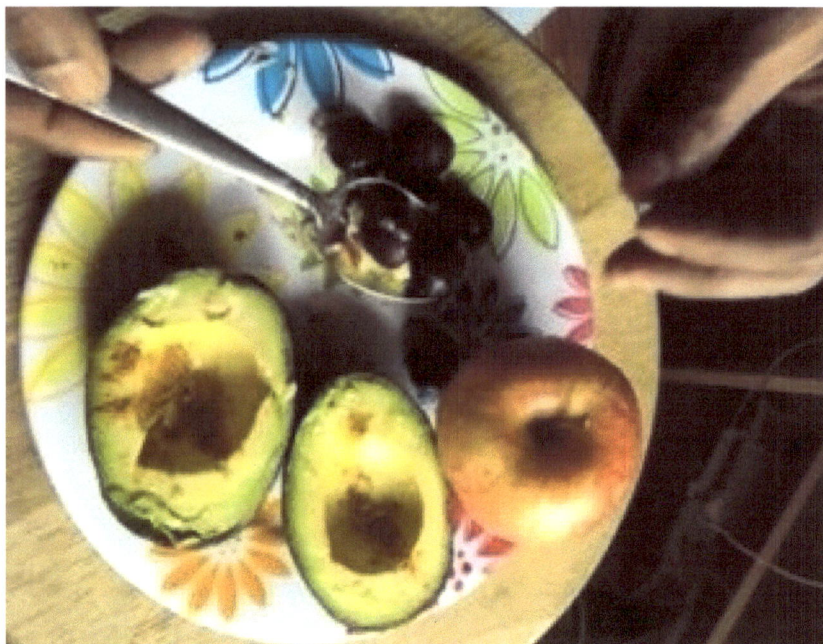

Avocados, apples and black beans

Heavy snack or small but hearty lunch

Sprinkle of Himalayan or Sea salt

½ teaspoon of turmeric

½ black pepper

1 teaspoon of olive oil or walnut oil

1 Apple

1 Avocado

Spoonful of black beans

Palm full of basmati rice

What you do not see here in the empty space is basmati rice. This meal is the perfect balance of fats, protein, carbohydrates and immune boosting spices. Surprisingly here we have a complete plant based protein with the black beans, avocado, apple and basmati rice. The immune boosting qualities of turmeric with black pepper and the 65 minerals and nutrients in Himalayan salt make this the perfect anytime meal not just a midday snack.

BASMATI RICE

	BROWN	WHITE
CARBS	33 G	37G
FATS	1.5 G	0
PROTEIN	4 G	3
DIETARY FIBER	2 G	0

CONTAINS OF 1/4 CUP

Note that basmati rice is a incomplete protein but can be completed with beans, whole grains and produce throughout the day

Roasted Pumpkin Seeds

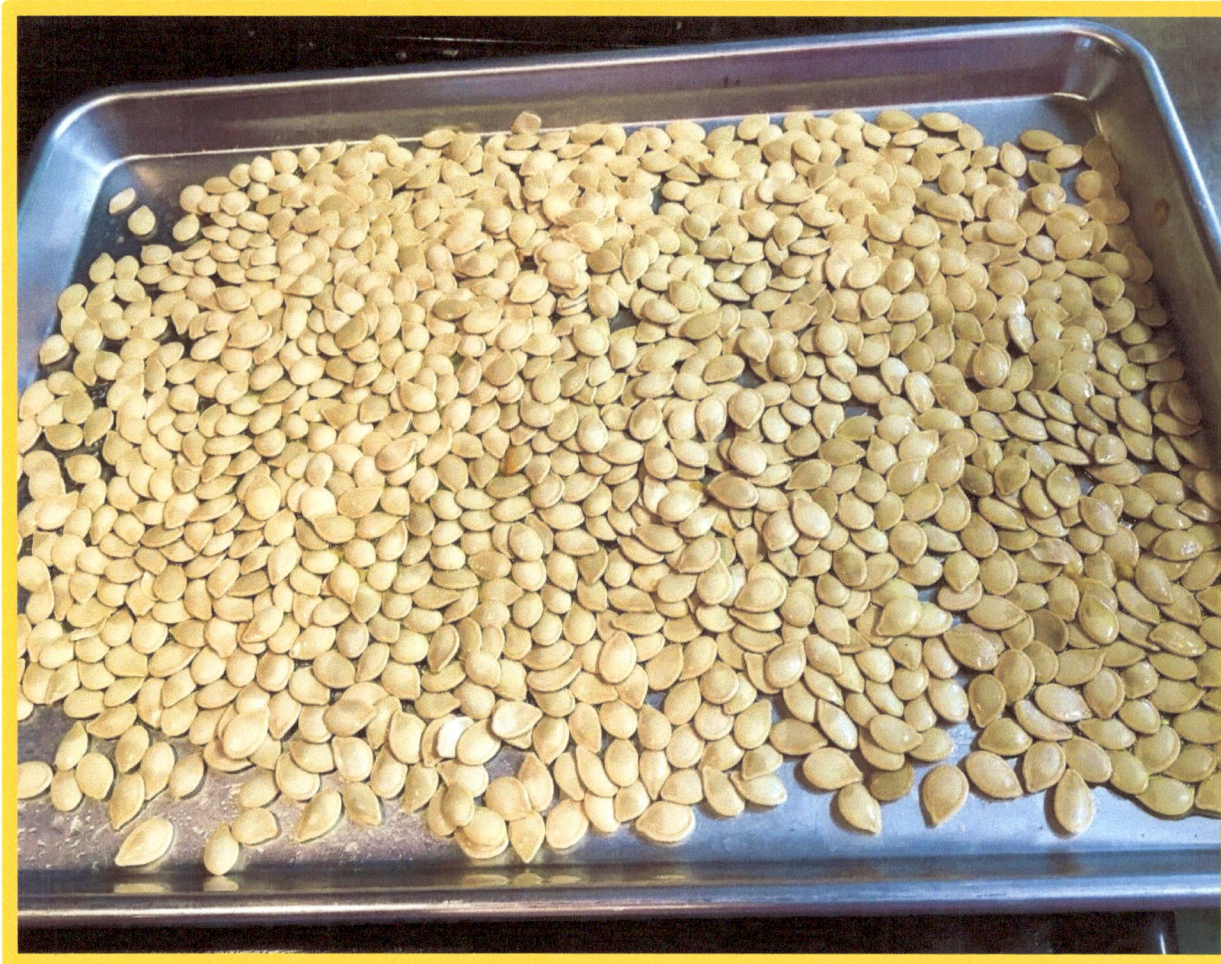

Pre-roasting

When we were preparing the pumpkins for baking, we decided to make a snack. So, we destringed and cleaned the seeds. After scooping out the baked meat we put the pumpkin skin or shell for composting. Ever part of the fruit was used and we helped the environment.

Spread pumpkin seeds evenly on a cooking sheet and drizzle 3 tablespoons olive oil. Bake on 400 F for 25 minutes or until golden brown.

Sprinkle with Himalayan salt (optional)

Enjoy!

Baked Apple Skins

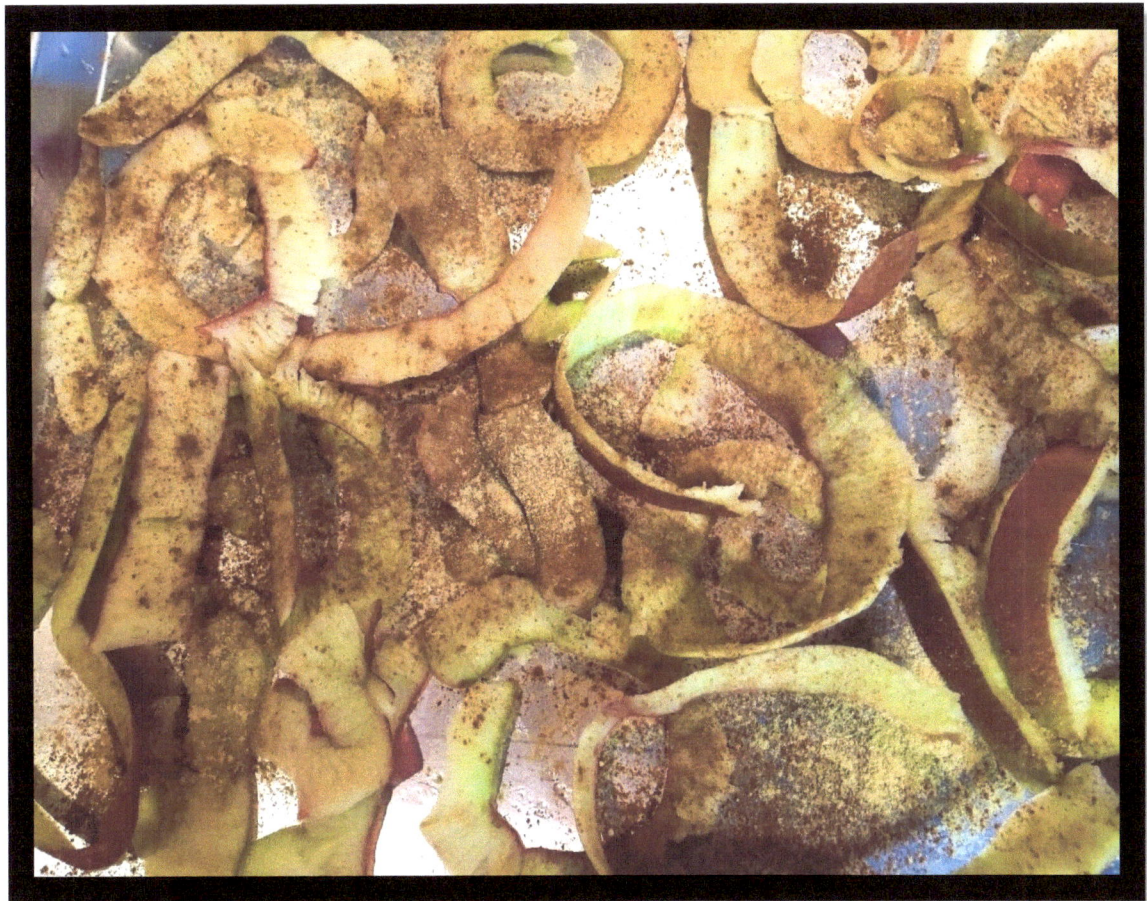

Ever make an apple pie and wonder what to do with all the skins? Less waste in cooking is a good practice. The apple core goes for composting; the meat for the pie and the skins for a snack.

Spread skins on a cookie sheet evenly. Sprinkle with cinnamon and ginger. Baked on 400 F for 20 – 25 minutes or until golden brown. These are a great chips alternative. This is generally a same day snack as they are so delicious they would not last long.

The same can be done with sweet potato skins or while potato skins. However, because white potatoes being on the dinner dozen you make reconsider eating them unless organic. Even then with caution.

DINNER

- VEGETABLES
- POULTRY
- FISH
- RED MEAT

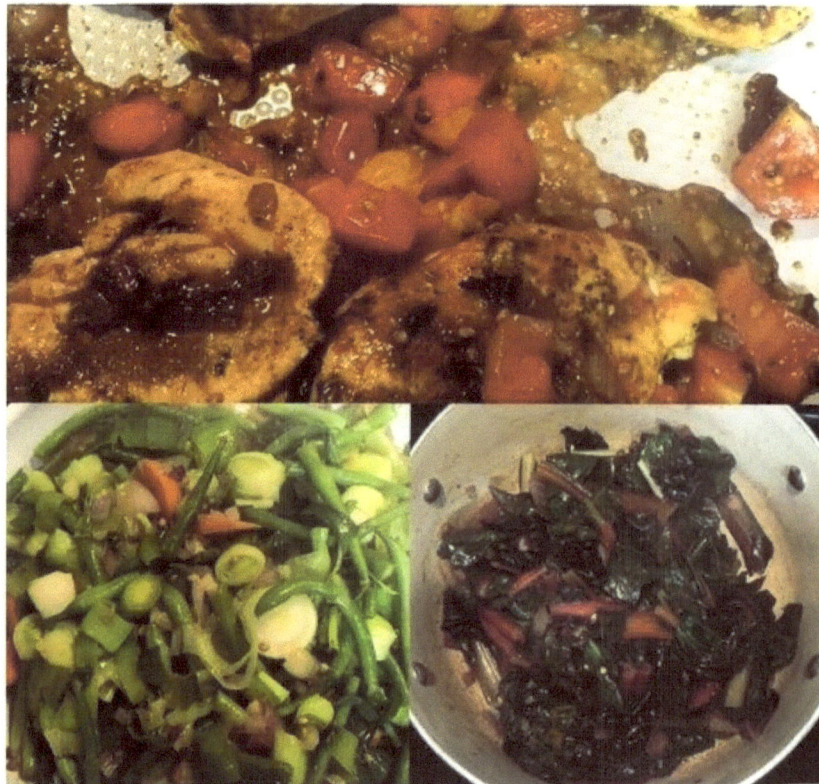

As we have seen the right vegetable combination can be a complete meal. We all know that we need to eat them but which ones should be staples and how can we used them as a source of protein. Then there are what spices to use? How much salt? Should I use salt?

In the next few pages I will cover, the few vegetables and legumes that I use as staples and how they fit into the protein equation and the important role that spices play in making vegetables more hearty.

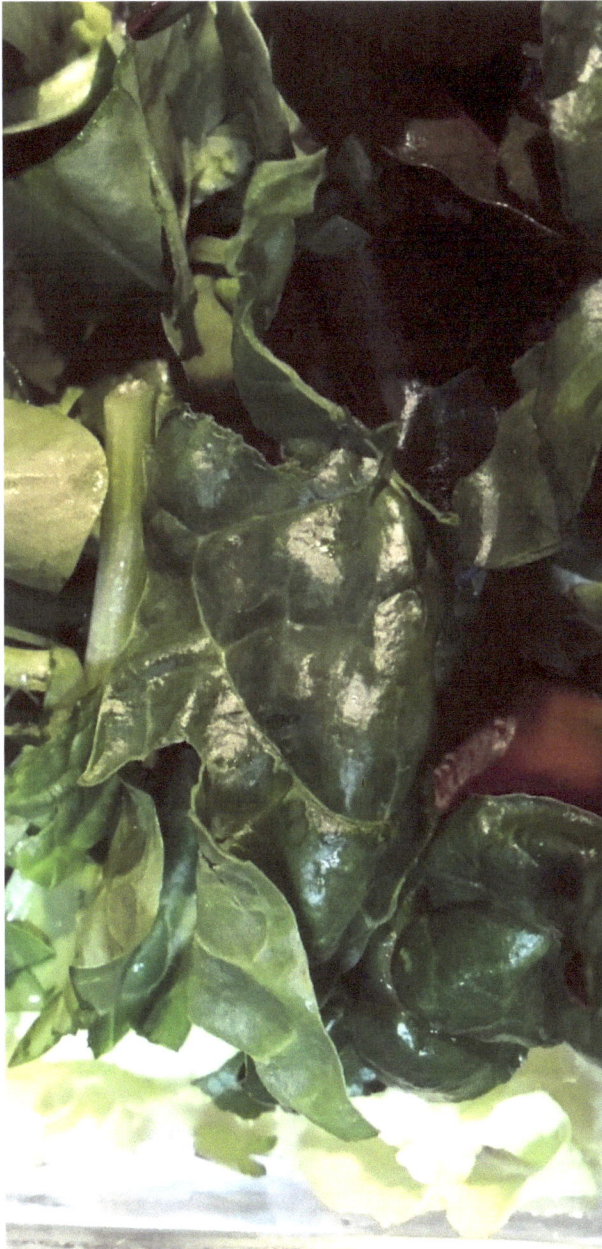

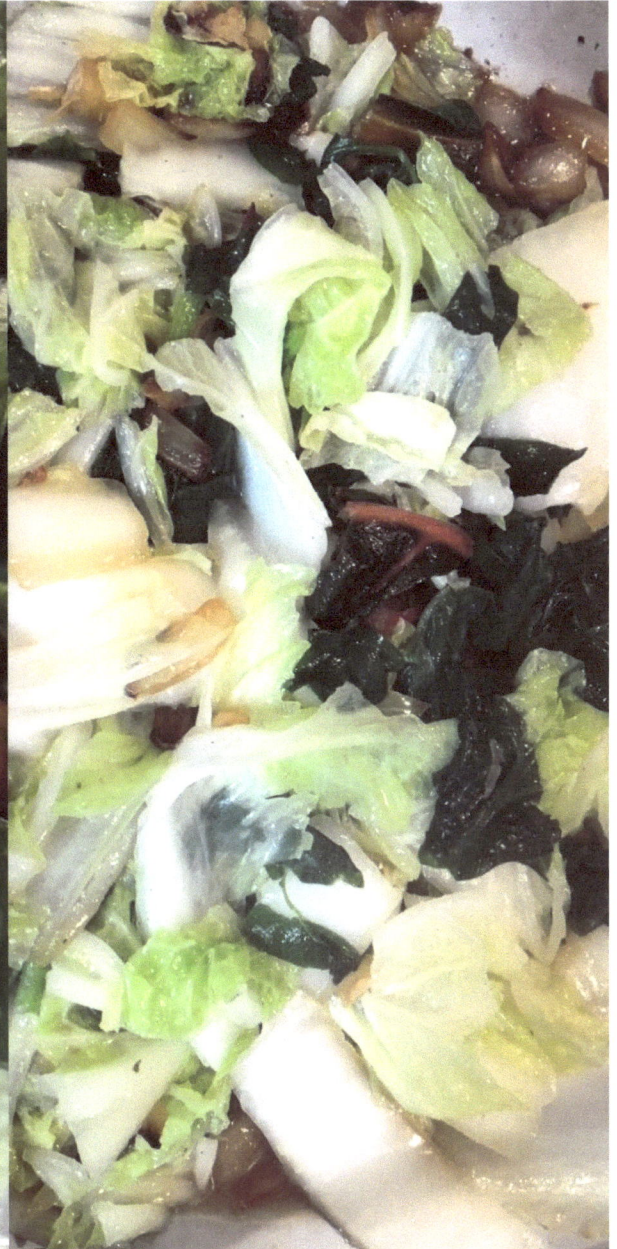

Before cooking   after cooking

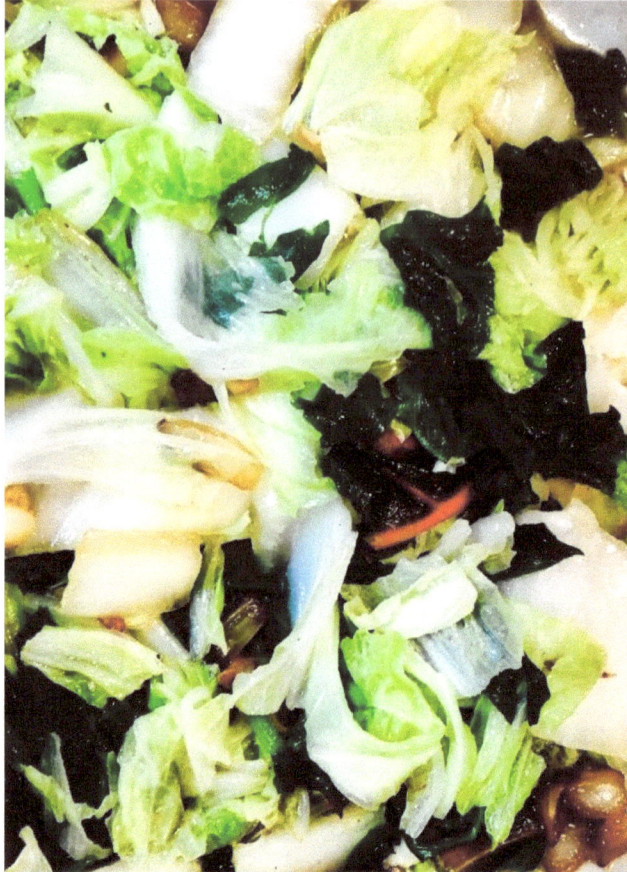

Full picture after 3 minutes of cooking

Steamed Sweet Greens

1 bunch of Rainbow Swiss Chard

½ a Napa cabbage

1 bunch of organic Tuscan kale

1 TSBP minced fresh ginger root

1 TSBP minced garlic

½ chopped red onion

1 TSBP of coconut oil

1 TSBP cumin seeds

Sauté ginger, onions, garlic in coconut oil for 2 minutes or until onions are golden. Wash and chop greens. Add greens to sauté stirring regularly. Sprinkle with Himalayan salt.

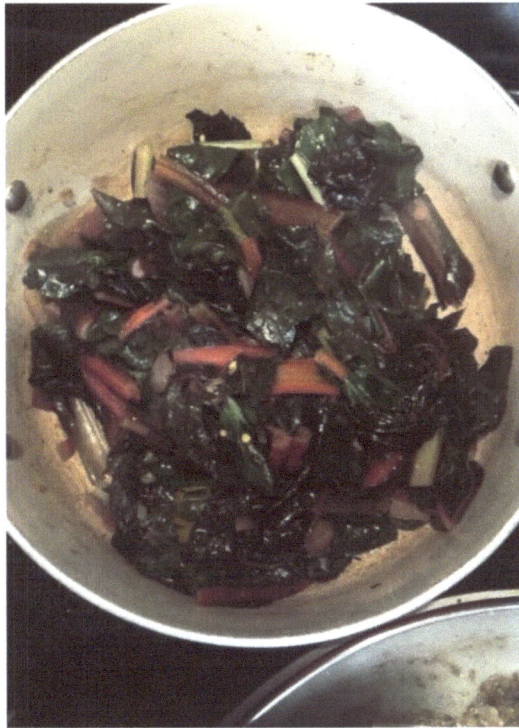

Bitter greens great substitute for Collard Greens 3 minutes

1 bunch of swiss chard

1 bunch dandelion

1 TSBP minced fresh ginger root

1 TSBP minced garlic

½ chopped red onion

1 TSBP of coconut oil

1 TSBP cumin seeds

Sauté ginger, onions, garlic in coconut oil for 2 minutes or until onions are golden. Wash and chop greens. Add greens to sauté stirring regularly. Sprinkle with Himalayan salt.

Note: This recipe can be doubled as needed.

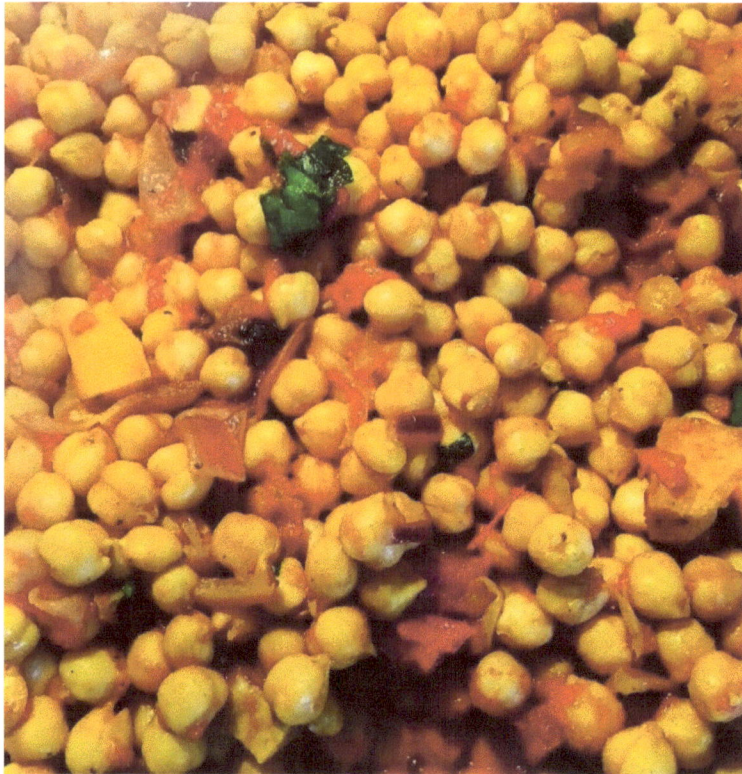

Sweet potato chick peas

1 large sweet potato   1 large tomato (optional)

29 oz can of organic chick peas or 1 lb. bag of dry chick peas

2 tsp turmeric

1 tsp cumin seeds

1 TSBP minced fresh ginger root

1 TSBP minced garlic

½ chopped red onion

2 TSBP of coconut oil

1 TSBP coriander powder

Directions:

- If using dry beans soak overnight.
- Sauté ginger, onions, cumin seeds garlic in coconut oil for 2 minutes or until onions are golden.
- Peel and chop potato into one inch cubes.
- Add garlic, chick peas and sweet potatoes.
- Stir every 5-8 minutes and add water ½ cup at a time if cooking with canned beans total cook time will be 20 minutes.
- If cooking with dry beans, do the sauté portion in the pan and then use the pressure cooker for the remaining time. Use the legume or beans setting.

This is a great replacement for using rice with beans and hearty enough to serve without meat. It can be complimented with a nice green salad or steamed bitter greens.

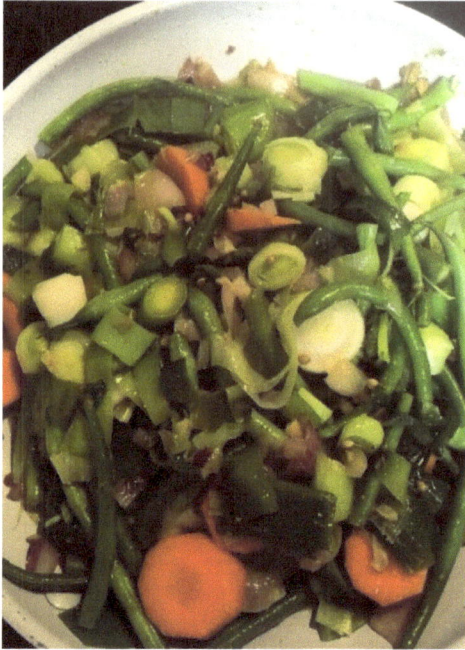

Leeks, Carrots and green beans (perfect balance of carbohydrates

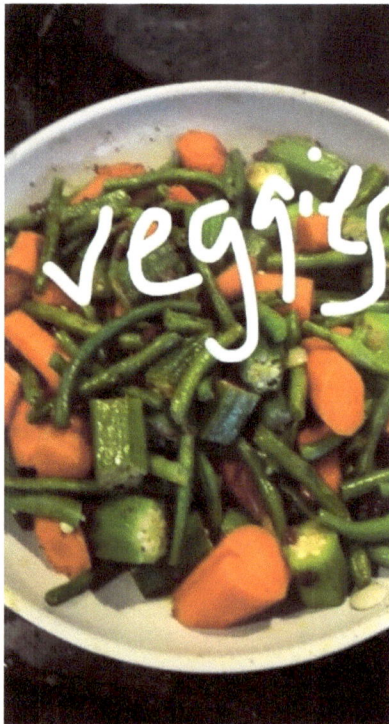

)

Carrots with leeks, okra or green beans, snow peas, Napa cabbage or bok choy are great options for slow digesting carbohydrates. Use them to replace paste or combined with certain types of rice can be a complete meal.

Cranberries are also another super food closely related to blueberries.

Prevent bacteria from sticking to the bladder

Help prevent bacteria from causing food-borne illness

May prevent tooth decay

Lowers LDL- cholesterol

Other anti-cancer properties

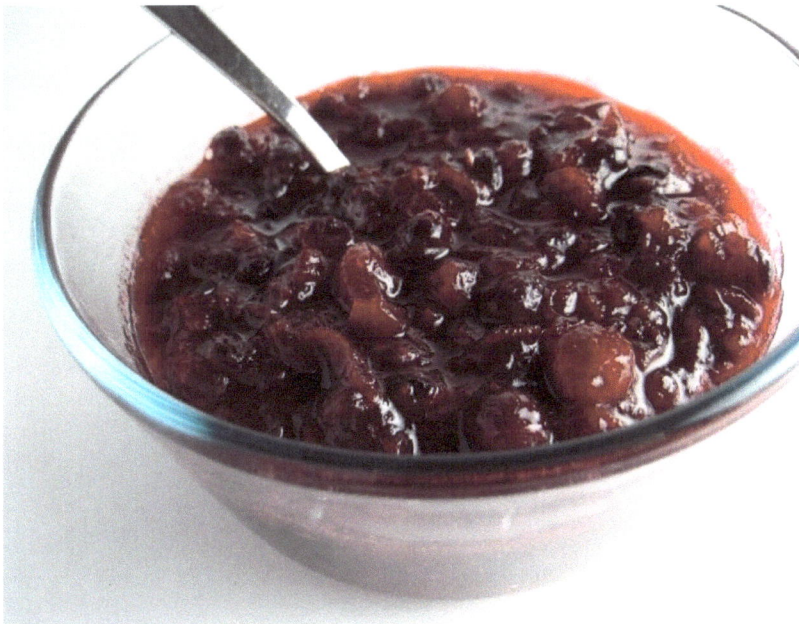

Cranberry sauce

1 bag of cranberries

1 cinnamon stick

2 cups of water

¼ cup of brown sugar

1 pomegranate

½ tangerine

Directions:

1. Bring water to a boil and add sugar.
2. Once the sugar has dissolved add cranberries, pomegranates, and cinnamon stick.
3. Cook on medium heat for 20 minutes or until it comes to a low boil.
4. Squeeze tangerine juice and throw in the zest or rind for added flavor and color.

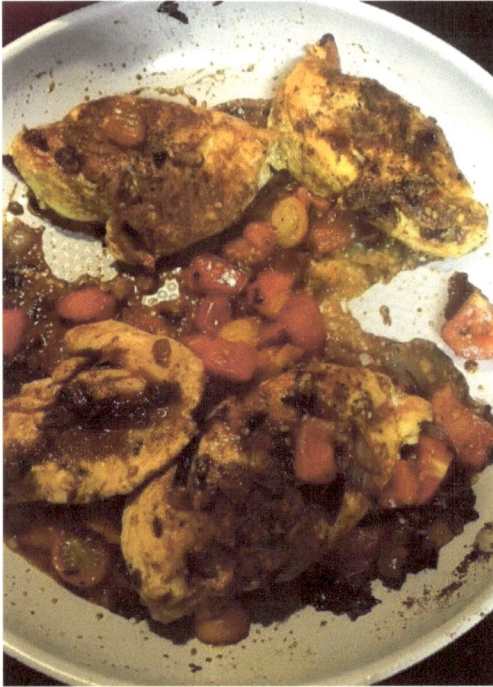

Curry chicken

- 3- pound chicken cuts into small pieces

- 1 TBSP Coriander powder

- 2 TBSP Turmeric powder

- 1 TBSP Paprika

- 1 large tomato

- ¾ bulb of garlic minced

- 1 red onion minced

- cilantro

- 1 TBSP Cumin seeds

- Dash Pink Himalayan salt

- 1 tsp Red pepper, 1 tsp Black pepper

- 1 TBSP ginger minced

Directions:

5. Clean and season chicken pieces with the spice mix.
6. Sauté onions and ginger with cumin seeds in 1 tablespoon of coconut oil add garlic right before adding chicken.
7. Chop up tomato and add in after chicken is brown.
8. Chop up cilantro and add.
9. Cook stirring often for 45 minutes or after 20 minutes' place in the pressure cooker for 40 minutes.

Serve with vegetables and rice. There is a section on suggested rice to eat and cook with lower glycemic values and higher nutritional value. Traditionally dal or lentils will also be served with chicken. You may also add potatoes, sweet potatoes or organic red potatoes.

Using the pressure cooker to complete the cooking process seals in the flavor and cooks out the extra fats.

Curry Salmon over Sweet Potatoes

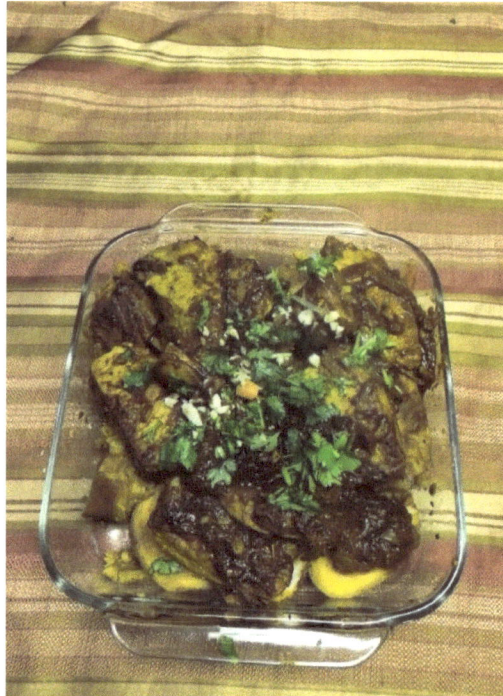

- 3 medium sweet potatoes or yams

- 1 TBSP Coriander powder

- 2 TBSP Turmeric powder

- 1 TBSP Paprika

- 1 tsp Clove

- ½ a green pepper

- 1 large tomato

- ¾ bulb of garlic

- cilantro

- 2 Salmon fillets skin on is fine

- 1 TBSP Cumin seeds

- Dash Pink Himalayan salt

- 1 tsp Red pepper, 1 tsp Black pepper

Directions

1. Clean and cut Salmon into several large cube pieces.

2. Clean and chopped tomatoes. Slice green pepper.

3. Mix cumin seeds and salt with tomatoes and green peppers.

4. Sauté tomato and green peppers in coconut oil until lightly browned.

5. Mince garlic and set aside.

6. Rub Salmon with spices mix and set aside.

7. Once tomatoes and green peppers are lightly browned sprinkle with ¾ of minced garlic.

8. Add one tablespoon of coconut oil to pan and the remaining garlic on low-medium heat. Spread throughout the saucepan.

9. Add salmon and brown on medium heat.

10. Flip over and brown the other side.

11. Add tomato and green pepper mix and ½ cup of water.

12. Put in pressure cooker for two minutes or put mix (fish, tomatoes and green peppers) in saucepan covered on low-simmer for ten minutes.

13. In the last minute add basil and then serve.

- Preparation Tip:

- Or same day in power pressure cooker

- Marinate fish before freezing

- Serving suggestion:

- Serve with a side of steamed in season vegetables or fresh salad

DESERT

- PIES
- COOKIES
- CAKES

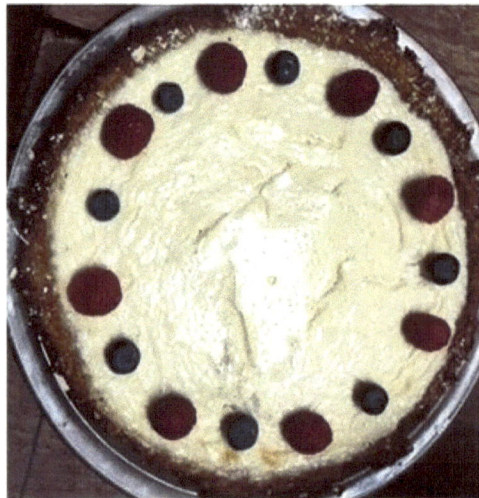

Before baking   *Baked Pumpkin*

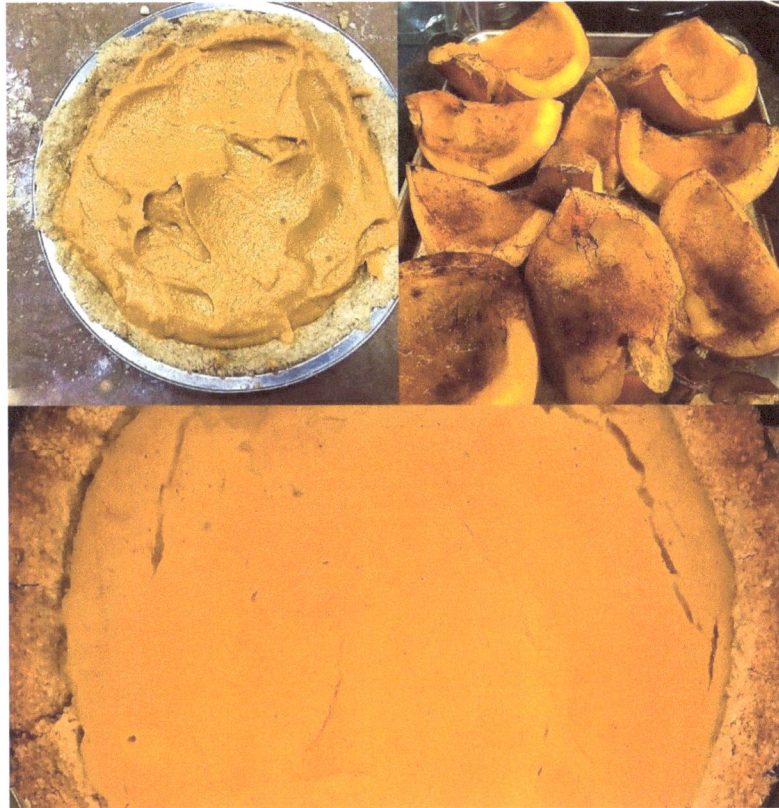

Fresh Pumpkin Pie

One of the best parts of fall is fresh pumpkin pie. Enjoy the experience to the fullest by going to the pumpkin patch and picking the pumpkin; clean them with the kids; cut and bake the pieces. Making your own puree, crust is a family bonding opportunity. Enjoy the process and breathe in all the memories that you create!

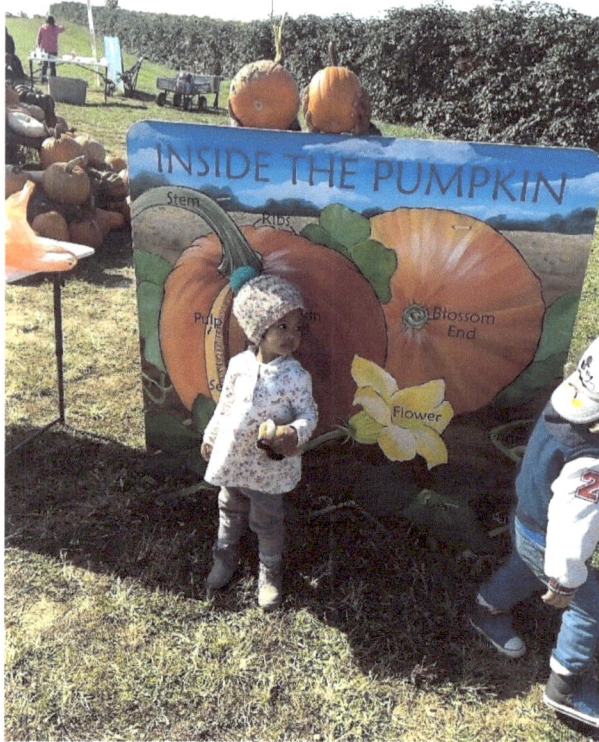

Arlene at the local pumpkin patch

Puree

2 small pumpkins (makes 4 cups)

2 cups of vanilla almond milk

¾ cup of brown sugar or maple syrup

2 tsp of cinnamon powder

1 tsp ginger powder or nutmeg

10. **Cut pumpkins into quarters and lather with coconut oil or olive oil.**
11. **Bake for 25 – 30 minutes on 400 F**
12. **The pieces should look as pictured above. Scoop out pulp and put in blender with brown sugar, spices and almond milk.**

Crust

4 cups of oatmeal

1 ½ sticks of cold real butter (can be grass-fed, Amish or organic)

3 TBSP of baking powder

2 tsp of cane sugar

½ cup of milk

3 TBSP of wheat flour

Parchment paper

Makes enough for a shallow or deep dish 8 – 9-inch pie pan.

1. *Blend the oatmeal in blender to a powder.*
2. *Dump into a large mixing bowl and mix well with baking powder and sugar.*
3. *Cut butter into cubes or slice into the powder mix.*
4. *Using a pastry masher or two butter knives, chop and mix butter into powder mix until fine pieces like biscuit dough.*
5. *Add milk and complete mixing by hand into a ball.*
6. *On parchment paper, spread flour and roll ball.*
7. *Start spreading the dough into the pie pan with three middle fingers from center to walls.*

No waiting fill in immediately with the puree. Bake on 375 F for 40 -45 minutes.

Apple Cobbler

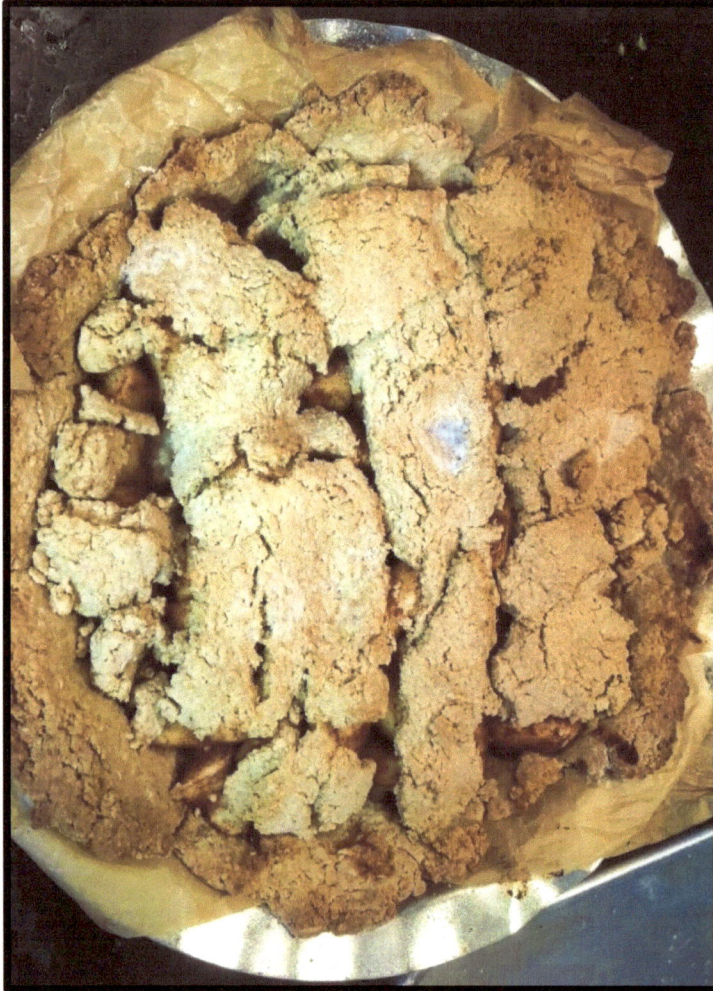

Interesting history on what is the difference between a pie and a cobbler. Most basic difference is that a cobbler has only one layer crust while pies often have full layers of crust. Also, a cobbler comes is various shapes, i.e. square, oval etc. whereas a pie is always round. Cobbler filing is beneath the dough layer and has no bottom dough. Finally, cobblers usually have a thicker biscuit like dough and less of a pastry like dough.

Why am I sharing this? Because I set out to make an apple cobbler and then made a pie because I thought they were the same. You and I both learned something new today. Now the next think you should know is that the crust I have created for this pie is more cobbler like but lighter. When you make, it you will understand or even if you make the pumpkin pie first, you will see the difference in the crust. Bon appetit!

Crust

4 cups of oatmeal

1 ½ sticks of cold real butter (can be grass-fed, Amish or organic)

3 TBSP of baking powder

2 tsp of cane sugar

½ cup of milk

3 TBSP of wheat flour

Parchment paper

Makes enough for a shallow or deep dish 8 – 9-inch pie pan.

1. **Blend the oatmeal in blender to a powder.**
2. **Dump into a large mixing bowl and mix well with baking powder and sugar.**
3. **Cut butter into cubes or slice into the powder mix.**
4. **Using a pastry masher or two butter knives, chop and mix butter into powder mix until fine pieces like biscuit dough.**
5. **Add milk and complete mixing by hand into a ball.**
6. **On parchment paper, spread flour and roll ball.**
7. **Start spreading the dough into the pie pan with three middle fingers from center to walls.**

> *Both apples remain firm during baking and will not breakdown like other apples varieties such as granny smith. Very sweet and intense flavor requiring less sugar.*

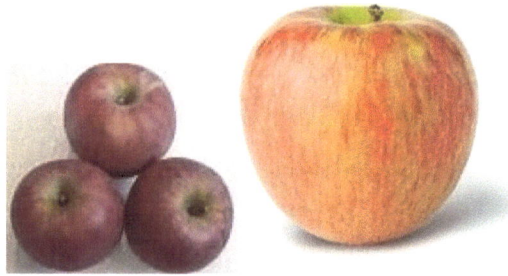

Winesap apples   Honeyscrip apple

Filling

7-8 Winesap or Honey crisp apples for natural sweetness peeled, cored, and sliced (peels for snacks, core for compost)

2 tsp of cinnamon

1 tsp ginger powder

1 tsp nutmeg

½ cup of brown sugar or maple syrup

¾ cup of water

1. *After apples, have been cored, peeled and sliced, place in a large bowl.*
2. *Mix with spices and sugar*
3. *Place parchment paper in the bottom of the pie pan and spread the dough from center to sides.*
4. *Pour the apples mix in the 8-9 inches cooking pan and pour the water evenly.*
5. *Place the crust on top of the apples*
6. *Skip step six if you are make a true cobbler with no bottom crust layer.*

Pie cooking instructions:

Cook for 25 minutes on 400 F covering the with parchment paper. Then remove the parchment paper and cook and additional 20 minutes on 375 F.

Cobbler cooking instructions

Cook for 40 minutes on 375 F covering with parchment paper. Then remove the last five minutes. If using glass, reduce time by five minutes.

Sweet Pumptato Pie and Tarts

Pumpkin and sweet potato   *Tarts in a muffin pan*

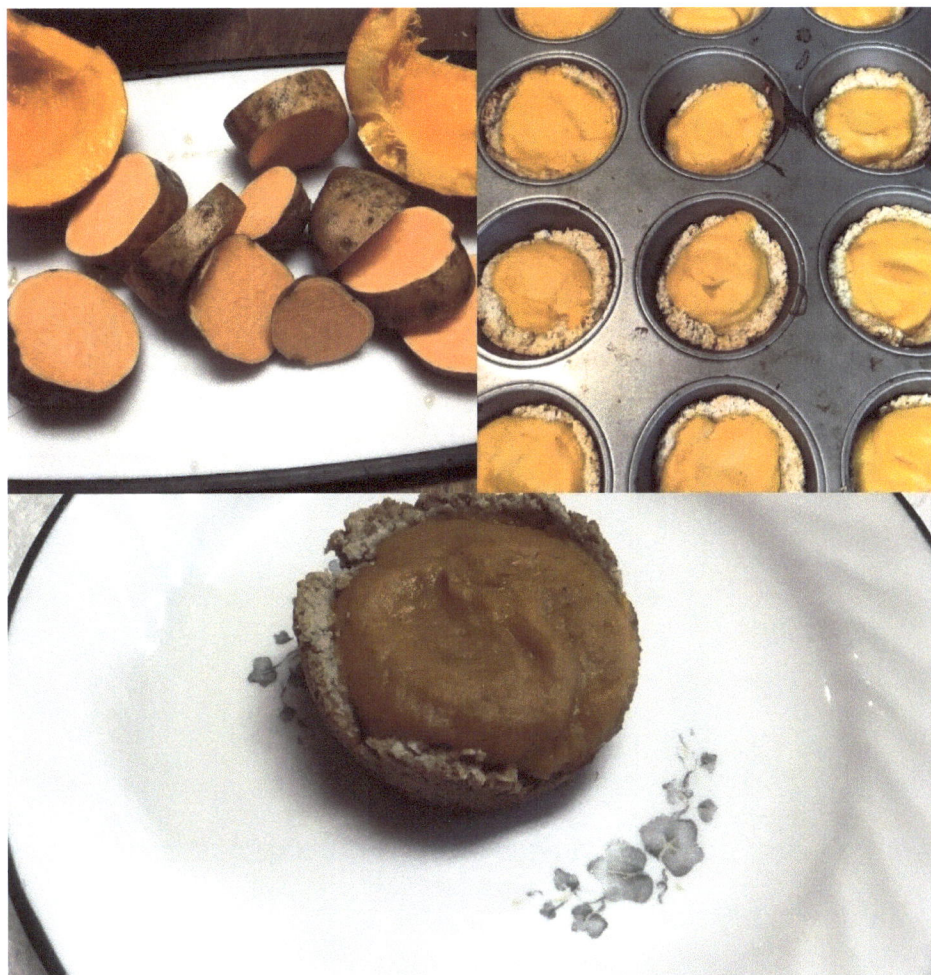

Sweet Pumptato Tart

You may be wondering what is a sweet pumptato pie or tart. It was what make when you have leftover sweet potato filing and pumpkin pie filing from making those two pies but not enough to make a whole pie of either. It was the invention of my daughter Muhibbah, she was helping me to make my pies and then we realized that we had leftover but not enough; so, she said, "Let's mix it together!" I thought was a great idea. "Then we can use less sugar because the sweet potatoes are naturally sweeter than pumpkin". That last part is not quite true. I say add maple syrup because it is sweeter than sugar and you can use less.

By now you can see that the crust recipe is the same for all my pies, so I will skip straight to the baking instructions. However, I will give the sweet potato filing recipe.

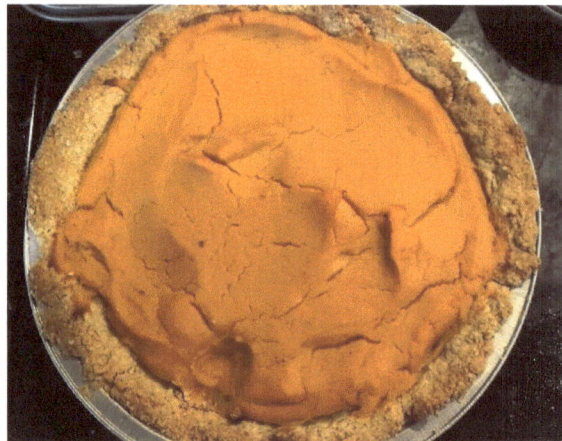

Sweet Potato Pie

Filing

4 large sweet potatoes (makes about 4 cups of puree)

2 ½ cups of almond milk

2 tsp cinnamon

2-3 TBSP brown sugar or maple syrup

2. **Clean and slice potatoes into 4 – 6 slices.**
3. **Place in power pressure cooker for 10 minutes or boil on stove top for longer.**
4. **Take off the skins and set aside for potato skin chips.**

5. *Sprinkle with cinnamon; mash and add sugar or syrup.*
6. *Place in blender or food processor for smoother texture and add almond milk. Blend until smoother not soupy.*

Using a muffin pan, place a small ball of crust mixture into each round and smooth from center to sides as you would with a pie dish. Add 2-3 tablespoons of filing and bake for 45 minutes on 375 F.

Oatmeal Cookies

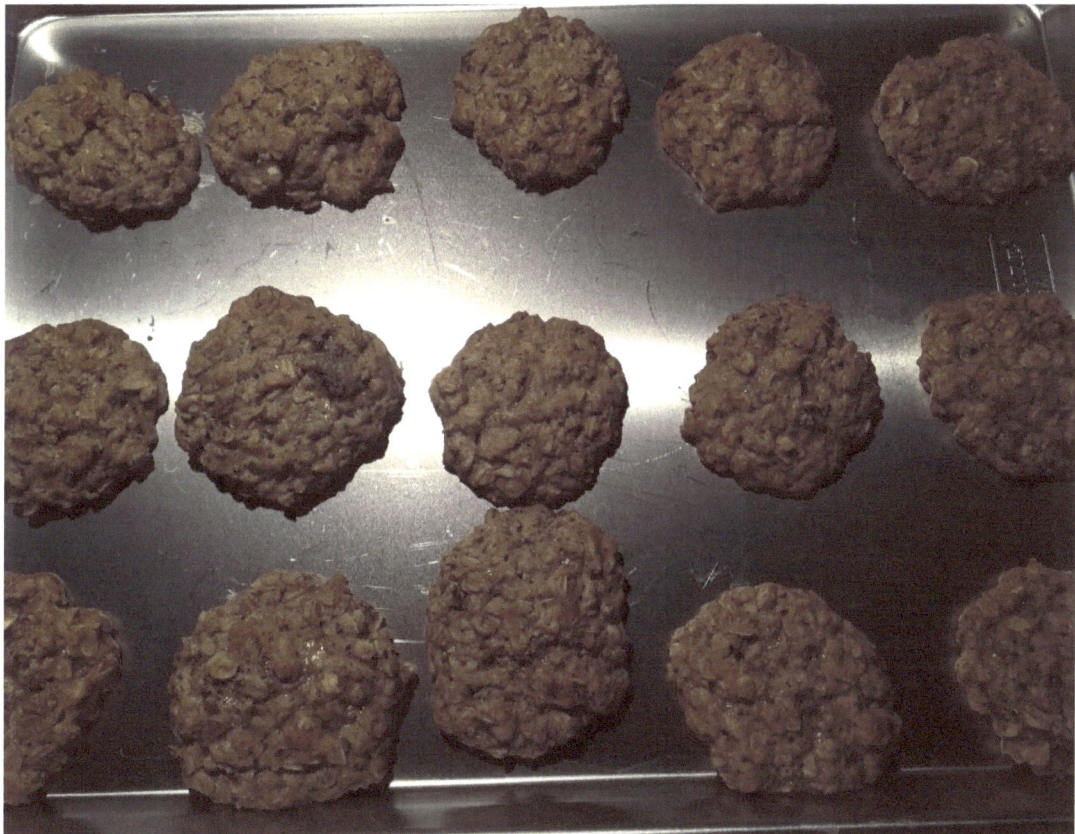

No childhood memory is complete without the smell and taste of oatmeal cookies. This recipe is adapted from Quaker Oats traditional recipe.

How about taking an old recipe and reducing the sugar and upping the protein? Instead of cacao nibs, golden berries or goji berries are also quite delicious. Play with the recipe and make it your own.

½ cup of cacao nibs

¼ cup walnuts, ¼ cup almonds

2 TBSP chia seeds

2 sticks of grass fed butter

3 cups of oatmeal

1 ½ cups of wheat flour

1 tsp of baking soda

½ salt (optional)

2 eggs

¾ cups of brown sugar, ½ cup of cane sugar

2 tsp cinnamon powder

1 tsp organic vanilla bean extract

Directions

1. Blend softened room temperature butter with sugars.
2. Mix flour, baking soda, cinnamon powder and salt together in a separate bowl.
3. Add eggs to the butter sugar mix one at a time until fluffy.
4. Fold in the wheat flour mixture until smooth.
5. Add in oats, nuts, chia seeds and nibs until smooth.
6. Scoop in 1 tablespoon sized balls placed an inch apart.
7. Bake for 14 minutes on 375 F.
8. Can also be made into bars by using a 13x9 in brownie pan and slicing.

Cheesecake

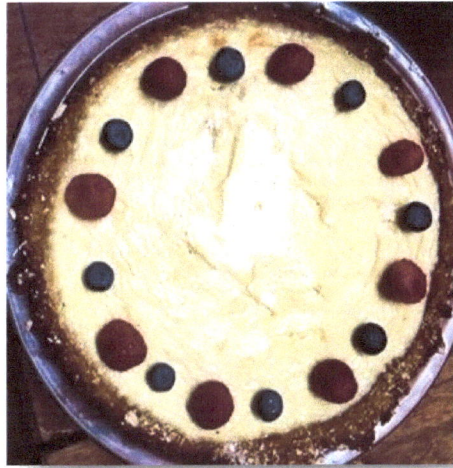

Crust

2 medium yams or sweet potatoes

1 cinnamon stick

1 TBSP coconut oil

¾ cup of blended oats

¼ cup blended nuts (walnuts, pistachios or almonds)

1. Bake yams or sweet potatoes. I use a pressure cooker with the ingredients listed and ½ cup water for ten minutes.
2. Blend oats and nuts.
3. Skin and mash potatoes into a paste. Blend in the oats and nuts mix.
4. Bake for ten minutes.

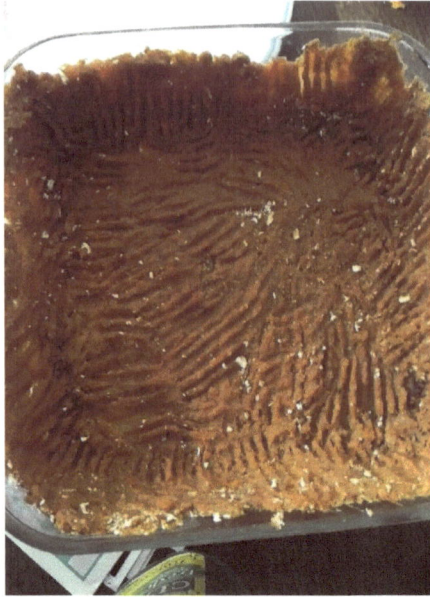

Filing

16 oz. of cream cheese

6 oz. of plain grass fed yogurt

1 cup of vanilla flavored grass fed yogurt

2 eggs

1. *Blend yogurt and cream cheese.*
2. *Add one egg at a time until creamy and fluffy.*
3. *Place in crust.*
4. *Bake for 35 minutes on 350 F.*

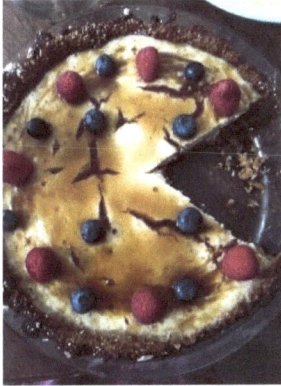

Topping Raspberries and blueberries or other in season fruit with Buckwheat honey

Brownie Delight

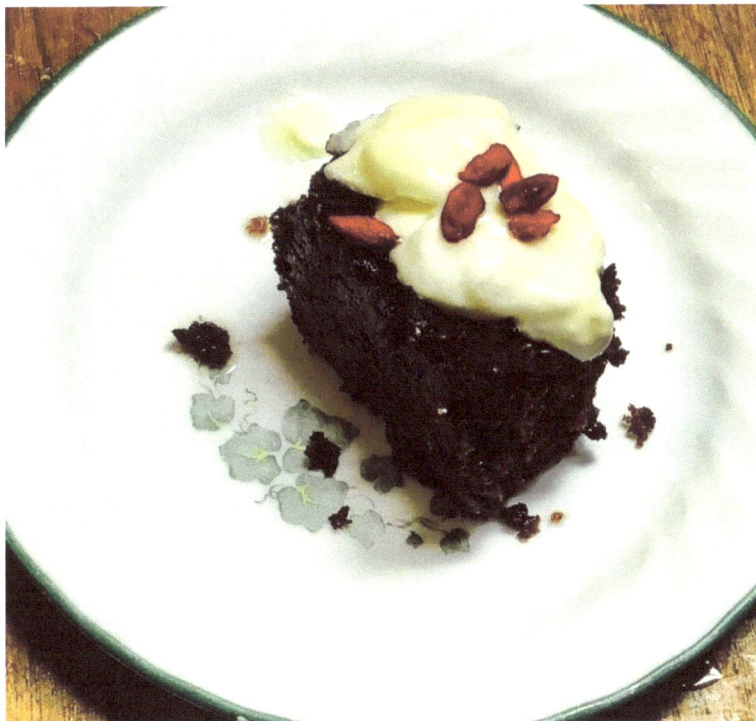

- *1 Cup* Chickpeas *(Garbanzo beans)* 15 oz. can - BPA free can liner

- *1/4 Cup* Grass Fed Butter, melted

- *2* Eggs

- *1/2 Cup* 100% Pure Maple Syrup *You can us honey as well*

- *2 Tsp* Pure Vanilla Extract

- *1/3 Cup* Organic Unsweetened Cocoa Powder *or Carob powder*

- *1/2 Tsp* Baking Powder

- *1 Pinch* Himalayan Salt

- *1/4 Cup Raw cacao nibs*

Adapted from 21- day fix brownies.

- *Preheat oven to 350 degrees*

- *Line a 9 x 9 backing pan with parchment paper. You can also use an 8 x 8 pan they will just be a little thicker and you might need to adjust the bake time*

- *Place chickpeas, butter(oil), eggs, maple syrup (honey) vanilla, cocoa powder, baking powder, and salt in a blender or a food processor. Blend or pulse to well blended*

- *Add in the chocolate chips and mix by hand*

- *Pour into your prepared pan and bake for 25-28 minutes or until a toothpick comes out clean*

- *Let cool completely before you cut them. It is quite decadent served warm.*

Holiday Bonus

Wild Rice

1 cup quinoa

1 cup parboiled rice

1 cup red rice

6 cups of water

1 stick of cinnamon

6 green cardamom

1 TBSP of fennel seed

1 TBSP coconut oil

Mix rice and quinoa together and wash. Add water, coconut oil and spices. Use a rice cooker or pressure cooker. Cook as directed by manufacturer.

This is a delightful treat both pleasing to the eye and palate. Nutrient rich red rice and light parboiled rice. In the following pages, you will see the nutritional values of parboiled and red rice and how it can be a replacement for stuffing. You may however, be familiar with quinoa. All three grains together add a powerful super power to your holiday meal accompanied with the bitter greens, cranberry sauce, sweet potatoes, carrots vegetable mixes and of course the turkey.

The final recipe is the turkey and its dripping gravy or "The Ungravy" as I like to name it. Basically, using the drippings of the turkey because of the spices all the work is done for you no need to add anything to enrich the flavor.

PARBOILED RICE

CARBS	41	G
NIACIN	4	MG
CALCIUM	30	MG
POTASSIUM	5	MG
IPROTEIN	6	G
MAGNESIUM		
ZINC		
FAT	5	G
DIETARY		
FIBER	4	G

CONTAINED IN 1 CUP

Note that because of the difference in processing it is a better source of fiber, calcium, potassium and vitamin b-6 than white rice. A glycemic score of 38 versus white rice at 89.

RED RICE

CARBS   87   G
FATS   4.9 G
PROTEIN   7   G
IRON   5.5 MG
ZINC   3.3 MG
POTASSIUM   256G
DIETARY
FIBER   10 G

CONTAINED IN 1 CUP

Research suggest that it may also lower cholesterol levels. It has a nutty flavor due to its thick hull and is mineral rich including trace amounts of magnese and sodium.

The Turkey and gravy

No holiday meal is complete without a turkey. It has such a distinct flavor that it often over powers most seasonings and spices. Over the years I have experimented with a variety of was to hold in the flavor and moisture. Most often the meat is literally falling off the bone. One way is to use an oven bake bag. Clean and marinate overnight. I like this because I can cook a 20- pound turkey in 2-3 hours.

The second way is to use a Turkey roaster. I prefer this option because you are not using plastic which can be harmful due to the estrogens.

Either way you will find a nutritious delicious treat in the seasoning and spices in the marinate.

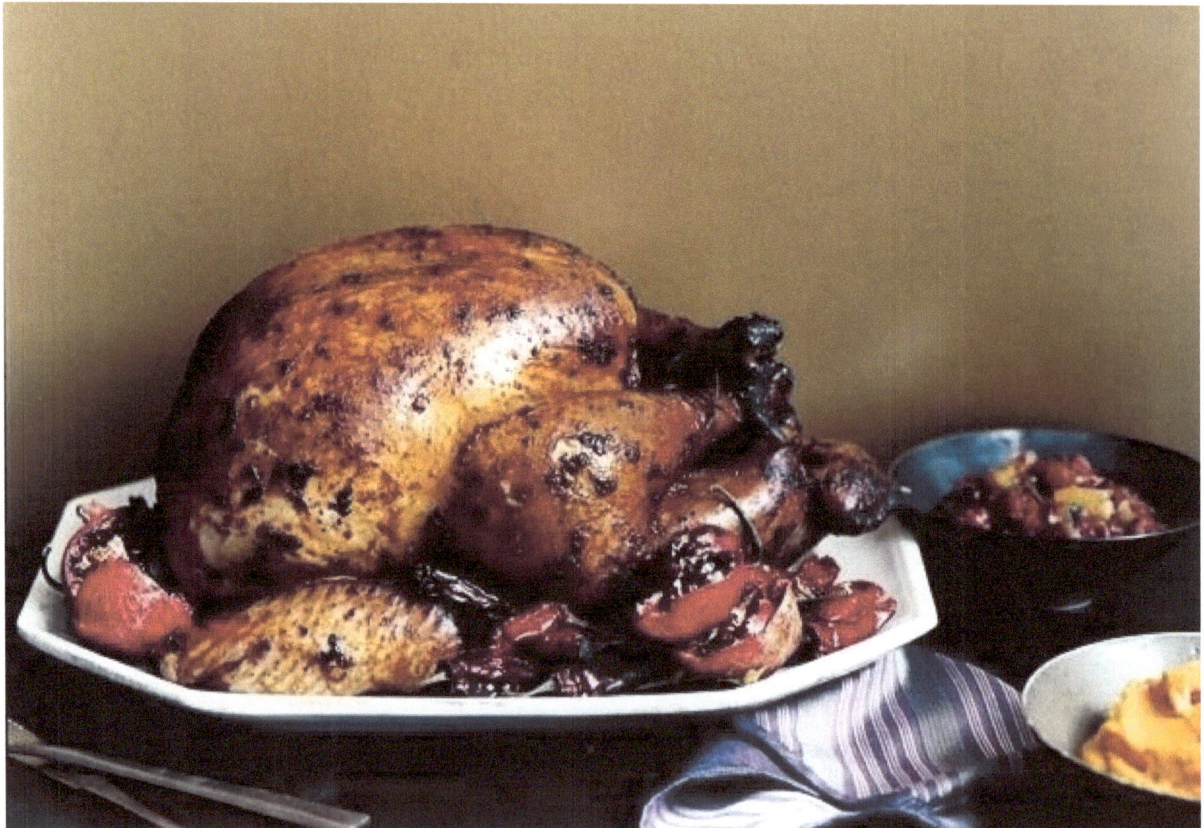

At the beginning of the recipe section, I included the garlic/ ginger paste and spice making recipes. It is always best to fresh toast low heat and grind your spices for optimum flavor. Always have a batch made.

To make the marinade first make the tandoori spice mix. The danger in purchasing prepackaged mixing are the sodium and possible lead content. All spices can be for at any Indian store.

Tandoori mix:

1 TBSP Coriander seeds

1 TBSP Cumin seeds

1 TBSP Whole black peppercorns

1 -3in cinnamon sticks broken into pieces

1 TBSP Cardamom seeds

1 tsp Fenugreek

1 tsp whole cloves

1 tsp chili powder

Toast for 2-3 minutes on low heat and grind.

Garam masala mix is less likely to be laden with sodium and can be purchased.

Marinade:

- 4 cups (1 quart) plain whole-milk yogurt
- 1/2 cup chopped peeled ginger
- 1/2 cup fresh lime juice
- 1/4 cup finely chopped garlic
- 1/4 cup paprika
- 2 tablespoons tandoori masala
- 2 tablespoons garam masala
- 2 teaspoons chili powder
- 1 teaspoon freshly ground black pepper

Turkey: 12 -14 pounds

- 1/4 cup Sea salt
- 5 black cardamom pods
- 5 green cardamom pods
- 1 tablespoon cumin seeds
- 1 medium red onion, chopped
- 2 celery stalks, chopped
- 4 garlic cloves

Directions:

Clean and wash well. Pat dry with a paper towel. Rub the turkey inside and out with marinade and place in the roasting pan overnight on its belly. The next morning take out of the refrigerator and let sit for an hour. Preheat oven to 400 F.

Salt the turkey and insert the above ingredients in the belly. Place the garlic strategically in the skin and neck. Cook in pan for 30 minutes and then lower heat to 350 F and cook for an additional 2.5 hours.

Let cool for at least 30 minutes and serve.

Drain the dripping and collect in a bowl to serve as the gravy. Enjoy!

Wishing you and your family health, happiness and peace always!

www.wordtherapypublishing.com

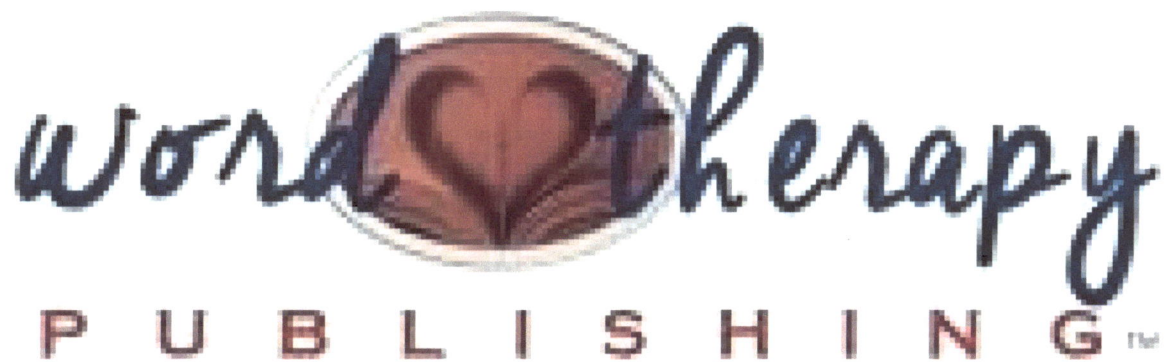

"A Message That Heals"